# FERTILITY MASSAGE FOR WOMEN:

Introducing The Malay Uterus Massage (M.U.M.)™

*Improving Women's Reproductive Health and Chances of Conception*

**SALWA SALIM**

Copyright © 2017 Salwa Salim

All rights reserved.

This book or any portion thereof may not be reproduced or used in any manner whatsoever without the express written permission of the publisher.

This book is not intended as a substitute for the medical advice of physicians. The reader should consult a physician in matters relating to her health, accordingly; particularly with respect to any symptoms that may require diagnosis or medical attention.

ISBN: 978-0-9989403-1-1

# **DEDICATION**

*To all the women out there trying to get pregnant.*

# *Table of* CONTENTS

Dedication ............................................................. iii

List Of Abbreviation............................................. vii

List Of Illustration................................................ ix

Preface..................................................................... x

Acknowledgments ............................................... xix

## PART I - Understanding Your Body ....................... 1
Chapter 1.1 - Introduction ..................................... 2

Chapter 1.2 - Mind & Body Connection .......... 12

Chapter 1.3 - Basic Anatomy & Functions of Female Internal Abdominal Organ................................. 19

Chapter 1.4 - Female Reproductive System .................. 24

Chapter 1.5 - Menstrual Cycle ........................................ 33

## PART II - History & Development of Massage & Fertility Around the World ..................................... 40
Chapter 2.1 - Massage in Traditional Medicine ............. 41

Chapter 2.2 - China ..................................................................48

Chapter 2.3 - Malay Archipelago
(Southeast Asia) ....................................................................53

Chapter 2.4 - Latin America ...............................................59

Chapter 2.5 - Japan................................................................61

Chapter 2.6 - Worldwide......................................................63

## PART III - Development Of Malay Uterus Massage™ by Salwa Salim, Uterus Heat Therapy & Vaginal Steam Therapy .......................................... 70

Chapter 3.1 - Malay Midwifery & Women's
Reproductive Health..............................................................71

Chapter 3.2 - Malay Uterus Massage™ by Salwa Salim,
Uterus Heat Therapy & Vaginal Steam Therapy............74

Chapter 3.3 - Practical Application....................................83

## PART IV - Benefits of M.U.M.™ Fertility Massage ................................................... 99

Chapter 4.1 - General Benefits......................................... 100

Chapter 4.2 - Uterus........................................................... 105

Chapter 4.3 - Ovaries......................................................... 112

Chapter 4.4 - Fallopian Tube............................................ 115

Chapter 4.5 - Surrounding Organs ................................. 117

Chapter 4.6 - Emotional Release ..................................... 120

## Part V Annex - Research Studies on Massage, Reproductive Health & Infertility in Women ..................................... 122

Massage Improves Pregnancy Rates and
Improves Successful IVF ................................................. 123

Massage Improves Women's
Reproductive Health ........................................................ 127

Relationship Between Stress and Infertility ................... 133

Relationship Between Relaxation
and Improved Fertility ..................................................... 139

Reducing Stress Through Massage ................................. 145

Glossary ............................................................................. 151

Bibliography ..................................................................... 154

Index .................................................................................. 166

About Author .................................................................... 174

# LIST OF ABBREVIATION

| ART | Assisted Reproductive Technology |
|---|---|
| ATMAT | Arvigo Technique of Mayan Abdominal Therapy |
| CAM | Complementary and Alternative Medicine |
| FBM™ | Fertile Body Model™ |
| FSH | Follicle Stimulating Hormones |
| IUI | Intrauterine Insemination |
| IUD | Intrauterine Device |
| IVF | In-Vitro Fertilization |
| LH | Luteinizing Hormones |
| NCAAM | National Center for Complimentary and Alternative Medicine |
| M.U.M.™ | Malay Uterus Massage™ |
| PID | Pelvic Inflammatory Diseases |

| **PCOS** | Polycystic Ovary Syndrome |
| --- | --- |
| **PMS** | Premenstrual Syndrome |
| **TCAM** | Traditional, Complimentary & Alternative Medicine |
| **TCM** | Traditional Chinese Medicine |
| **WHO** | World Health Organization |

# LIST OF ILLUSTRATION

Fig 1: South East Asia (Malay Archipelago) Map

Fig 2: Fertile Body Model™

Fig 3: Basic Anatomy of Female Internal Abdominal Organ (Anterior View)

Fig 4: Female Reproductive System (Sagittal View)

Fig 5: Female Reproductive System (Anterior View)

Fig 6: Ligaments in Female Reproductive System (Superior View)

Fig 7: Menstruation Cycle Chart

Fig 8: Body Landmarks


Table 1: The Four Seasons of the Menstrual Cycle

Table 2: 28 Days Menstrual Cycle Sample based on The Four Seasons of the Menstrual Cycle

# PREFACE

My journey into the world of fertility started from my professional working experience as a medical sonographer, where I routinely encountered women with infertility issues. My encounters with these women sparked my interest in understanding their condition, as well as their efforts to seek available treatment options, even those beyond medical solution. I started gathering information from different sources and discovered a whole new world of holistic, natural treatment in treating infertility; some backed by research studies, while others were just old wives' tales and remedies.

The viable option in treating infertility using natural treatments, in the category of traditional, complementary or alternative medicine (TCAM), is such a huge discipline that it was necessary to choose a specialization for me to explore. With that, I decided to delve into my personal interest, which is massage. There are limited literature published linking the effectiveness of massage to women's reproductive health. These findings were very recent and results were promising. In my opinion, this subject area is

## Fertility Massage for Women

still underdeveloped and has a great research potential. With new groundbreaking studies in this field, a more natural, affordable, safe and effective solution could be developed for infertility; thus, I embarked on an intensive learning journey traveling far and wide across the world, attending courses and trainings related to massage and fertility.

My studies and travels included informal learning from midwives and healers. Interestingly, my research brought me back to my roots, and the answer was much closer than I had anticipated. I found myself in the deep, rural villages in Penang, Malaysia, where my earliest childhood memories of a *kampong* remain. This was an intimate connection to me, as it was the village my mother grew up in. I was told that my late great-grandmother was the *mak bidan kampung*, a village midwife coming from generations of midwives and healers. Her skill in the arts of traditional massage was passed down to my mother, which she still practices today. Where my journey led me was enthralling. Although my educational background and work experience has been inclined towards Western medicine, the solution I was seeking for was in my heritage. It came to no surprise that regardless of how far I had professionally pursued the mainstream medical and healthcare route, I had eventually returned to my roots to relearn traditional massage as part of a healing treatment. As the Malay saying goes, *dalam keturunan*, which roughly translates to "it's in the lineage". My mother mentioned how this was passed down the family line, and it was only a matter of time before I took an interest in it.

The Art of Malay traditional medicine is still very much practiced today, even amongst the non-Malays in this region. According to World Health Organization (WHO) Traditional Medicine Strategy (2014 - 2023) Report, the demand for such services will continue to increase [1]. I made it my personal goal to do further research in this field in order to bridge the knowledge and practical skills of the Malay traditional medicine, specifically in the areas of women's health and massage, to be worldly recognized as part of TCAM. In 2014, Mummy's Fertility massage program was set up in Singapore to provide natural fertility services for women, where we perform the Malay Uterus Massage™ (M.U.M.) by Salwa Salim as part of our fertility program. The program was very well received from women of different cultural groups and walks of life. The results have been very satisfactory.

M.U.M.™ is a specific massage technique, as part

---

[1] World Health Organisation (WHO). (2013).WHO Traditional Medicine Strategy, 2014-2023. *Hong Kong, China: World Health Organization*, Retrieve from:
http://apps.who.int/iris/bitstream/10665/92455/1/9789241506090_eng.pdf

## Fertility Massage for Women

of the Malay massage practices performed on women for improved reproductive health. With this, my team and I developed this technique further and standardized it as a practice. The team consisted of Malay women in their 50s and 60s, with at least 10 – 40 years of experience in the field. They have personal experiences and training from either an apprenticeship from *tukang urut* (traditional massage therapist) or acquired the art that was passed down from their teachers, grandmothers, mothers or aunts. "Malay" refers to the race of people found in the Malay Archipelago, which geographically stretches from Brunei, East Timor, Indonesia (excluding western New Guinea) Malaysia, Philippines, and Singapore[2]; however, for the purpose of relating this to the development of M.U.M.™ techniques, "Malay" here comprises of traditional practices found in Singapore, Malaysia, Brunei and partly Indonesia. Another point to note is the word "uterus" is synonymous to "womb" which refers to the anatomical structure of a particular part of the female reproductive system. Similarly in the Malay language, uterus has at least five different terms; thus,

---

[2] Reid A. (2001). Understanding Melayu (Malay) as a Source of Diverse Modern Identities, *Journal of Southeast Asian Studies,* 32, 295 - 313

this book may use these terms: "uterus massage" and "womb massage" interchangeably.

In my journey of discovering different natural treatments of infertility, I met some of the most inspiring individuals who are experts in their own field. All of them have a common goal of helping couples conceive. With their credible backgrounds, either supported by studies or success stories, I manage to collaborate with them and incorporate these different natural treatments into Mummy's Fertility Program. During my consultations with my clients, I personally encourage women to be more conscientious and proactive in improving their health and wellness. I created the **Fertile Body Model**™ where I advocate practicing a holistic approach to not only address any physical and physiological dysfunction in their bodies, but also improve their state of mind. This is extremely important to create a fertile environment in their bodies necessary for conception and pregnancy; what I describe as a *fertile body*.

In order to achieve a *fertile body*, I advise women to undergo lifestyle changes, requiring them to make diligent decisions in their everyday life. One is to remove themselves from toxic environments that may be harmful to their fertility health, such as heavy chemicals, heavy metals, pesticides, radiation, etc.; and eliminate bad habits, such as smoking and excessive coffee or alcohol consumption. The other way is to incorporate healthy lifestyle changes such as, improving nutritional intake by following a recommended diet and use of supplements; attaining a healthy, physical body with massage, yoga and exercise; creating a hormonal balance in their body with castor oil, aromatherapy essential oils and massage; nurturing a healthy mind and body connection with better stress management, sufficient sleep, yoga, meditation and counselling; and understanding their body rhythm through charting their mensuration cycle using the body basal temperature and cervical mucus method, and beginning a regime of regular fertility massage to improve fertility, and many more.

Although some of these approaches may seem to have minimal impact individually, combining all these different methods may increase chances for a successful conception. After all, even if all these techniques failed in directly helping a woman conceive, nothing is wasted as she will still benefit from a healthier body and mind.

Please note that this book is not meant to replace the knowledge and care of a licensed medical practitioner. This book aims to educate the general readers, especially Mummy's Fertility clients, to better understand what M.U.M.™ is and the conditions to improve fertility. Mummy's Fertility Program can help increase the overall chances of conception as a standalone practice, or in conjunction with any other programs that does not intervene or contradict with our program.

Our program was created specifically to help women with infertility, menstrual, menopausal and postnatal issues. Not only do we have many success stories of women becoming mothers (naturally or with assisted conception), Mummy's Fertility Program has also helped many women with regulating menstrual cycles, relieving menstrual symptoms, relieving menopausal symptoms, reliving abdominal discomfort, and reducing postnatal recovery time and symptoms.

My team and I are continuously improving our program. We hope, like many women out there whom we have helped to realize their dreams of motherhood, you too will find our program useful, or at least find this book enriching. I wish you all the best in putting in a conscientious effort in doing what you can to improve your chances of pregnancy and achieving a full-term pregnancy, as well as being blessed with the gifts of health and motherhood.

With Love & Light,

*Salwa Salim*

Salwa Salim
Women's Reproductive Health Expert

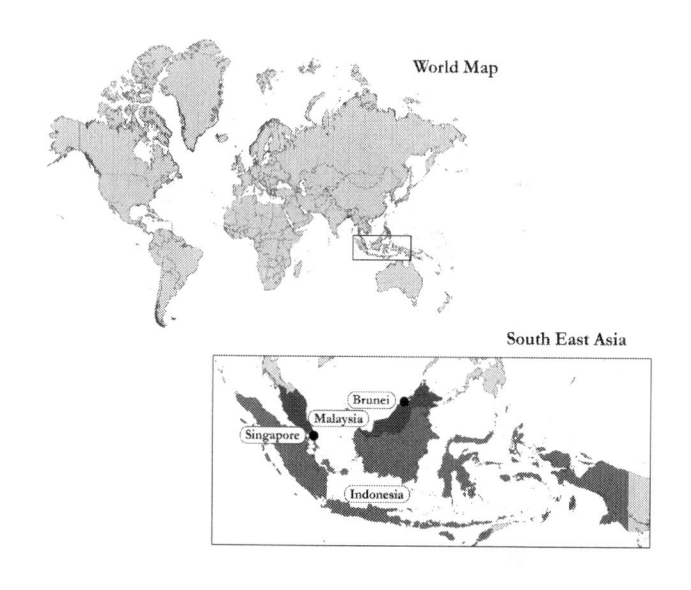

**Fig 1:** South East Asia (Malay Archipelago) Map

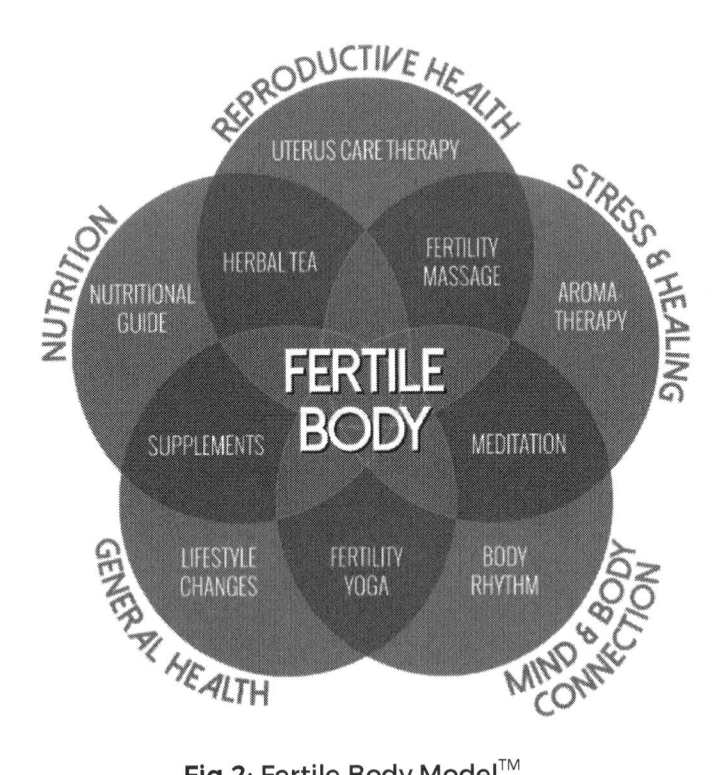

**Fig 2:** Fertile Body Model™

# ACKNOWLEDGMENTS

Most importantly, I want to express my immense appreciation to my mother who is my Chief Massage Therapist, popularly known as Mama Gie. Her heritage, skills, knowledge and support have encouraged me to write this book and preserve the Malay traditional healing practices. I would also like to acknowledge and extend my heartfelt gratitude to all the *makcik urut* who has contributed or imparted their invaluable knowledge and skills to me, in one way or another.

A formal thank you to my editor who advised me with the direction of the book, to my illustrators, as well as all the authors mentioned in the bibliography page for their contribution to this book.

To my clients, who have given me the motivation to write this book, I thank you all for giving me your support and having faith in me. You have become an integral part of my life through your stories and allowing me to share your joy of motherhood.

Salwa Salim

To my then fiancé, now husband and father to my child, who kept encouraging me why I should persevere and reminding me how much my work could help realize many women's dreams of motherhood.

And especially Adam and Aaren, who are my stress-relievers, yet at times are the very source of my stress.

# PART I

UNDERSTANDING YOUR BODY

# CHAPTER 1.1

## Introduction

Infertility is a disease of the reproductive system defined by the failure to achieve a clinical pregnancy after 12 months or more of regular, unprotected sexual intercourse[3]. For women, infertility can be described as the inability of a woman of childbearing age to become pregnant, maintain a pregnancy, or, carry a pregnancy to live birth. Infertility in women can be categorized either as primary infertility, where a women fails to achieve pregnancy, or secondary

---

[3] F. Zegers-Hochschild et al. (2009). International Committee For Monitoring Assisted Reproductive Technology (ICMART) And The World Health Organization (WHO) Revised Glossary Of ART Terminology, 2009, *Fertility And Sterility* 92, no. 5: 1520-1524, 1522.

## Fertility Massage for Women

fertility where a woman fails to achieve pregnancy again following a previous pregnancy. Female infertility issues affects up to 48.5 million women worldwide, with statistics showing that the numbers are most prevalent in South Asia, Sub-Saharan Africa, North Africa/Middle East, Central Eastern Europe and Central Asia[4].

Hence, it is important to understand what it takes to create a *fertile body* (conducive fertile environment) in the female body with the right conditions for pregnancy to happen. To highlight the importance of this, I created an analogy of the female body in preparation for conception through the stages of pregnancy:

> "Imagine the female body to be the most complex *machine* ever existed responsible for the productions of humans. With just a fusion of a sperm and an egg, this *machine* multiplies and differentiates the cells, assembling themselves into bones, nerves, organs, muscles, skin and blood with such an intricate and complex design.

---

[4] Maya N. Mascarenhas et al. (2012). National, Regional, And Global Trends In Infertility Prevalence Since 1990: A Systematic Analysis Of 277 Health Surveys', *Plos Med* 9, no. 12 (2012): e1001356.

This is carefully timed in a systemized convoluted production for 9 months. With such a critical task, shouldn't this *machine* undergoes regular maintenance to ensure all the parts of the *machine* are working perfectly in order to manufacture the *product*?"

It is important for the whole of the female body to be at its optimal health during the preconception period in order to prepare for a successful conception and pregnancy. Female infertility is more than just a case of dysfunctional reproductive organs or related hormones. It could also be an indirect cause of physical or physiological dysfunction in a non-related part of the body. Aside from that, the mental and emotional well-being may also be the inhibiting factor to conception.

Hence my approach to achieve this optimal fertile environment in the female body is through improving the overall health and well-being of the female body through natural methods. I advocate a holistic natural approach mentioned in the earlier section through nutrition, herbs and supplements, exercise, yoga, meditation, aromatherapy, etc. Having mentioned this, the aim of this book is to introduce fertility massage, namely our signature method of M.U.M.™ by Salwa Salim, to be accepted as part of a natural treatment regime. We explain what M.U.M.™ is and highlight how

## Fertility Massage for Women

this method may be effective in increasing the chances of conception.

Before we move on, let us take a look at the causes of female infertility and where M.U.M.™ can fit as a treatment. Medical studies have shown that approximately 40% of all infertility cases are due to the male factor, with the next 40% due to female factors, and the rest of the 20% are due to a condition known as unexplained infertility. Mechanical and hormonal problems account for up to 90% of the female factor, including cervical problems, uterine factors, tubal diseases or blockages, peritoneal issues like endometrium, and failure to ovulate amongst some of the more commons ones[5].

The first option is usually to seek medical advice for a viable treatment. This includes safe and effective hormonal treatments using medication to induce ovulation for those with ovulatory problems, surgical procedure if the cause of the interference is a physical obstruction such as tubal diseases or blockages,

---

[5] Mumford, K. (2004). The stress response, psychoeducational interventions and assisted reproduction technology treatment outcomes: A meta-analytic review. (Graduate Theses and Dissertation, University of South Florida, Scholar Commons, 2004), 32 – 27.

endometriosis or fibroids, artificial insemination by introducing the sperm directly into the cervix or uterus, and assisted reproductive technology where the egg and sperm are manipulated outside the body before reintroduced back into the uterus, the most common procedure In-Vitro Fertilization (IVF).

But what if the treatment options available are not suitable or affordable for all women? These treatment options do not come without a hefty price tag. Hormonal treatments, for example, may have a relatively high success rate, but the side effects make them unfavorable, ranging from mild to severe cases of nausea, bloating, mood swings, hot flushes, headaches, pelvic discomfort and weight gain, to just name a few[6].

What about the rest of the women experiencing unexplained infertility? If a medically fit and healthy woman of childbearing age is unable to become pregnant, what can be done about it? Artificial

---

[6] American Society for Reproductive Medicine. (2012). Medication for inducing ovulation, Patient Information Series, *American Society for Reproductive Medicine*. Retrieved from:
http://www.asrm.org/uploadedFiles/ASRM_Content/Resources/Patient_Resources/Fact_Sheets_and_Info_Booklets/ovulation_drugs.pdf, 8-9.

## Fertility Massage for Women

insemination, or assisted reproductive technology, may be the solution if all else fails, even though it is an invasive, painful, and expensive procedure. Even so, the success rate for intrauterine insemination (IUI) for example, is only 5-20%, and IVF is 40% at most, which is also subjected to the age and health of the women during the procedure[7].

If the objective of a woman considering the options above is to get pregnant, then her efforts should not be restricted to just medical intervention if alternative solutions offer a safe and effective method that can either be a standalone solution or works in conjunction with the medical intervention mentioned above. Some of the available treatments that can be found around the world include acupuncture, mind-body therapy, hypnosis, yoga and massage. Some of these methods have proven research studies on how it can directly or indirectly help with infertility issues, while many others, such as M.U.M.™ have assimilated research studies done, and are working towards getting support and funds to substantiate their findings, considering the

---

[7] Resolve.org, (2015), What Are My Chances Of Success With IVF?, *RESOLVE: The National Infertility Association,* Retrieve from: http://www.resolve.org/family-building-options/ivf-art/what-are-my-chances-of-success-with-ivf.htm

good track record of success stories coming from testimonials of clients.

To understand how M.U.M™ can be developed to be a treatment option for infertility issues in women, we will take a look at the history, development, benefits and practical application.

Depending on the condition, M.U.M.™ has the ability to address some of the medical conditions above: i) as a sole treatment, for example massage is the only non-invasive alternative treatment for blocked fallopian tubes due to an adhesion or scarring[8]; ii) in conjunction with the medical treatments above, for example massage on the abdomen has been researched to improve success rates of IVF[9]; iii) as aids in the management of infertility or its side effects or symptoms, for example, stress is a major inhibiting factor for infertility[10]; where massage is

---

[8] Wurn, B., Wurn, L., Roscow, A., King, R., Heuer, M., & et al. (2004). Treating female infertility and improving IVF pregnancy rates with a manual physical therapy technique, *MedGenMed*, *6*(2), 51.

[9] Wurn, B., Wurn, L., Roscow, A., King, R., Heuer, M., & et al. (2004). Treating female infertility and improving IVF pregnancy rates with a manual physical therapy technique, *MedGenMed*, *6*(2), 51.

[10] Domar, A. D. (2007). Coping with the Stress of Infertility, Fact Sheet Series, Fact Sheet 15, Infertility & Stress. *RESOLVE: The National Infertility Association*, Retrieve from: http://familybuilding.resolve.org/site/DocServer/15_Coping_with_

a form of relaxation technique that could lower the stress and anxiety levels associated with infertility[11][12].

Massage is an ancient remedy practiced worldwide for thousands of years to treat all sorts of ailments and illnesses[13]. Massage has been noted to address infertility issues for both men and women, where methods have been proven successful. However, the success of fertility massage has never been properly and comprehensively documented, published or widely available.

Massage for infertility issues is considered a specialization, or a subset of massage therapies available for both men and women, focused on improving their reproductive systems respectively. As massage is done by hand, the therapist deploys different basic massage techniques including

---

the_Stress_of_Infertility.pdf?docID=5705

[11] Valiani M. et al. (2005). The Effect of Relaxation Techniques to Ease The Stress In Infertile Women, *Iranian Journal of Nursing and Midwifery Research*, 15 no. 4: 259.

[12] Field T. et al. (2005) Cortisol decreases and serotonin and dopamine increase following massage therapy. *Int J Neurosci* 115, no. 10 (2005): 1397-1413.

[13] Mumford, K. (2004). The stress response, psychoeducational interventions and assisted reproduction technology treatment outcomes: A meta-analytic review.

effleurage, petrissage, kneading, rubbing and friction to stimulate the skin, muscles, ligaments, bone structures, internal abdominal organs or even on the reproductive organs itself.

The focus is usually on the reproductive organs and the immediate surrounding muscles, ligaments, structures and organs that are in close proximity, especially the upper and lower abdomen, pelvis and sacrum. The general rule is to massage these areas to loosen all the tightness in the muscles and ligaments that may cut off the blood circulation, or any organs or structures that may affect or impede the regular function of the reproductive system. The massage is also common at non-specific sites of the body.

As with any massage, the general benefits include increased circulation, reduced fluid retention, strengthened immunity by improving lymphatic drainage, strengthening of muscles, reduced tension, stress relief and alleviating depression. Additionally, for women, massage helps the realignment of the uterus back to its original position, management of painful periods, regulation of hormones, restoration of regular ovulation cycles, and breaking down the adhesions in the uterus. Stimulating the ovaries helps with the hormonal production aim at restoring the functions of the whole reproductive system.

## Fertility Massage for Women

As we explore the topic further, you will understand how massage has been a prevalent form of treatment found independently all over the world, in different cultures, dated back to the ancient times and is still very much relevant and applicable today.

# CHAPTER 1.2

## Mind & Body Connection

In the introduction, I mentioned that infertility issues are not necessarily a physical or physiological condition since 20% of infertility issues in women are unexplained[14]. Some medical practitioners dispute the idea of unexplained infertility by claiming that it is a false diagnosis, where diagnostic tools used to determine the infertility issues have failed to reveal a credible underlying cause for their condition. These women were diagnosed with unexplained infertility by default; where actual clinical

---

[14] Domar, A. D. (2015c). What truly is the relationship between stress and IVF outcome?, *The Domar Center for Mind & Body Health*. Retrieve from: www.domarcenter.com/blog/2011/03/what-truly-is-the-relationship-between-stress-and-ivf-outcome-2/

problems exist, but the root of infertility remains unknown. Most other views point to unexplained infertility in women as a condition that is associated with the mind and body.

Considering a physically healthy woman who is medically fit, but with an unexplained infertility, it is likely that this is linked to her mental or emotional state. There are direct causative links of mental and emotional states on the body. In the early 20th century, Wilhelm Reich, an Austrian psychoanalyst who pioneered the subject of human psychoanalysis, discovered the mind-body connection as the foundation to human psychoanalysis. This is the basis of many studies showing the relationship of stress, or negative feelings, or unexpressed emotions like anguish, guilt, shame and low self-esteem to infertility issues[15][16].

Reich discussed in his book Character Analysis, how the physical body stores the emotional or mental stress, tension, or trauma a person experienced throughout his or her life. When the negative experiences are not

---

[15] Clay, R. (2006). Does stress hinder conception? The relationship between mental state and fertility is a complex one. *American Psychological Association,37 (8)*. Retrieved from: http://www.apa.org/monitor/sep06/stress.aspx

[16] Reich, W. (1972). *Character Analysis*. New York: Farrar, Straus and Giroux.

managed well, the body will attempt what Reich terms "armoring" to protect the body from further harm. Over the years, if these emotions are not addressed and resolved, they will eventually reveal themselves in our postures. According to Reich, patterns of "armoring" include high, tight shoulders; slouched, hunched shoulders; chin stuck out; deflated chest; and widening or narrowing of the eyes[17].

Reich suggests that if a person has the ability to allow him or herself the freedom of physical expression, he or she believes that person will be able to empower him or her by choosing emotions and actions in life, as this affects the conditions of the body. Although Reich has experimented with radical ways of slapping, pinching, and twisting parts of his subject's body to get rid of negative emotions trapped in the subject's body, he recommends a more subtle approach to expelling negative emotions in the body through massage therapy. With massage, the body releases emotional tensions that especially dwell in areas like the shoulders, chest, and abdomen to allow healing. I personally experienced clients who were in the midst of their massage sessions suddenly bursting into tears, then feeling lighter afterwards. We all hold some form of emotional strews in our body, and according to

---

[17] Domar, *Coping With The Stress Of Infertility*.

Reich, massage gives relief that the body needs.

The mind is inextricably linked and inseparable to the body, where one or the other cannot be neglected to achieve optimal health. This involves the psychological, or mental, emotional and spiritual state. Alice Domar, a psychologist specializing in mind-body therapy for infertility, states that mind-body techniques include both physical skills, such as relaxation techniques, and physiological techniques as cognitive restructuring, social support, coping with negative emotions, as anger, guilt and self-nurturance[18].

To create a *fertile body* through optimal health, issues need to be addressed concurrently or independently to increase the overall chances of pregnancy. Our reproductive organs are very sensitive, as it can choose to shut down if it is not functioning optimally to save the body's health[19]; therefore, in order to restore the health and vitality of the reproductive organs, it is crucial to examine all areas of a person's life, including her physical, emotional and spiritual needs.

---

[18] Clare, B. (2015). *Fertility massage therapy* (1st ed.). Mayfair, London: Fertility Massage Therapy & Training.

[19] Lewis H.R. & Lewis M.E. (1972). *Psychosomatics: How Your Emotions Can Damage Your Health* New York, Viking Press.

To demonstrate this, a study done by Howard and Martha Lewis (1972) highlights how the subconscious mind can affect conception. They did a case study on a woman who had a fear of pregnancy complications and the birthing process. During tests, her doctor discovered that the muscles surrounding her fallopian tube involuntarily contract during ovulation; thus, blocking the sperm from reaching the egg. Her doctor commented on the phenomenon saying, "An emotional crisis or shock may close these tubes just as it may make one clench fist"[20].

A study done by Yale University (1985) focuses on the importance of emotional issues that could interfere with conception. The results showed that the group undergone therapy to address their infertility issues had a 60% conception rate compared to the control group of only 11%[21]. Another study by Wasser, Sewall and Soules (1993) also found that psychosocial distress contributes significantly to infertility, which may be an

---

[20] Sarrel, P., & DeCherney, A. (1985). Psychotherapeutic intervention for treatment of couples with secondary infertility, *Fertility and Sterility, 43*(6), 897-900.

[21] Wasser, S., Sewall, G., & Soules, M. (1993). Psychosocial stress as a cause of infertility, *Fertility and Sterility, 59*(3), 685-689.

important factor in cases of unexplained infertility[22].

These studies indicate how the mind and body connection is very powerful in determining the state of fertility in an individual. It is crucial to give as much attention to the mental and emotional, as well as the physical condition of a person, which points to the necessity of reducing stress, depression and anxiety through the practice of massage. Massage has always been known to induce relaxation, where many studies have proven how massage can reduce anxiety and depression in individuals[23][24]. A study published in the Journal of Psychosomatic Research (1993) revealed that the IVF success rate is dependent on the mood of the individual, which proved that women suffering from depression have less than half the success rate of conception[25]. This

---

[22] Hou W. et al. (2010). Treatment Effects of Massage Therapy In Depressed People, *The Journal of Clinical Psychiatry*. 71 no. 7 (2010): 894-901.

[23] Mayor, C. A., Rounds, J., & Hannum, J. (2005). A meta-analysis of massage therapy research. *Psychological Bulletin, 130*(1), 3-18

[24] P. Thiering, J. Beaurepaire, M. Jones, et al., "Mood State as a Predict Treatment Outcome After in vitro fertilization. emrbyo transfer technology (IVF/ ET)", Journal of Psychosomatic Research 37 (1993): 481-491.

[25] P. Thiering et al., "Mood State as a Predict Treatment Outcome After in vitro fertilization. emrbyo transfer technology (IVF/ ET)"

itself is a persuasive reason why massage should be performed in addition to fertility treatments, where numerous studies have shown the benefits of how relaxation helps reduce infertility in infertile women[26].

---

[26] Valiani et al. *The Effect Of Relaxation Techniques To Ease The Stress In Infertile Women.*

# CHAPTER 1.3

## Basic Anatomy & Functions of Female Internal Abdominal Organ

The female reproductive system is directly affected by the neighbouring internal abdominal organs. It is important to understand the functions and locations of these internal organs and how they are positioned in relative to the reproductive system and how their functions could affect the reproductive system either directly or indirectly. This chapter will give an overview of the basic anatomy of the female internal organ.

**Large Intestines:** The portion of the intestine that extends from the ileum to the anus, forming an arch around the convolutions of the small intestine and including the cecum, colon, rectum and anal canal. It is also called large bowel.

**Liver:** The largest gland of the body lying beneath the diaphragm in the upper right portion of the abdominal cavity. It secretes bile that is active in the formation of certain blood proteins, and in the metabolism of carbohydrates, fats and proteins.

**Ovary:** One of the paired female reproductive organs that produce ova and certain sex hormones, including estrogen.

**Small Intestines:** The narrow and winding upper segment of the intestines, also known as the small bowel. This is the organ where digestion takes place and most of the nutrients are absorbed by the blood.

**Stomach:** The enlarged sac-like portion of the digestive tract between the esophagus and small intestine, lying just beneath the diaphragm.

**Urinary Bladder:** A muscular membranous elastic organ located in the anterior of the pelvic cavity that temporarily holds the urine.

**Uterus:** A hollow muscular organ consisting of a body, fundus, isthmus, and cervix located in the pelvic cavity of female mammals where the fertilized egg implants and develops into the fetus.

Fertility Massage for Women

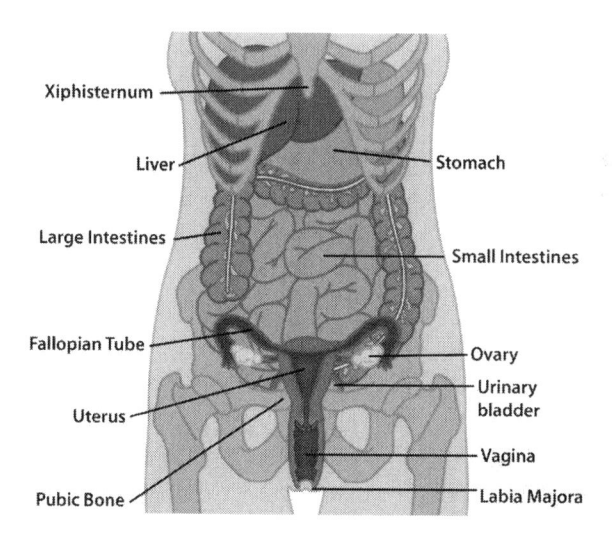

**Fig 3**: Basic Anatomy of Female Internal Abdominal Organ (Anterior View)

## Additional Information of Organs Directly Adjacent to Uterus

**Large Intestines:** The large intestines (colon and rectum), part of the digestive system, have the function of absorbing water. It is the area where solid waste is collected and stored before eventually passing through the anus as waste material. This structure lays behind the uterus cervix and vagina. Similar to the bladder, if the uterus is out of position or if uterus expands (during pregnancy), pressure is placed on the large intestines causing constipation.

**Urinary Bladder:** The bladder is an elastic organ located directly below the uterus, sitting on the pelvic floor. If the uterus is out of position or if uterus expands (during menstruation or during pregnancy) the bladder is pushed downwards, which may decrease the urine capacity in the bladder, causing frequent urination.

Source: The American Heritage® Medical Dictionary. (2007)

Fertility Massage for Women

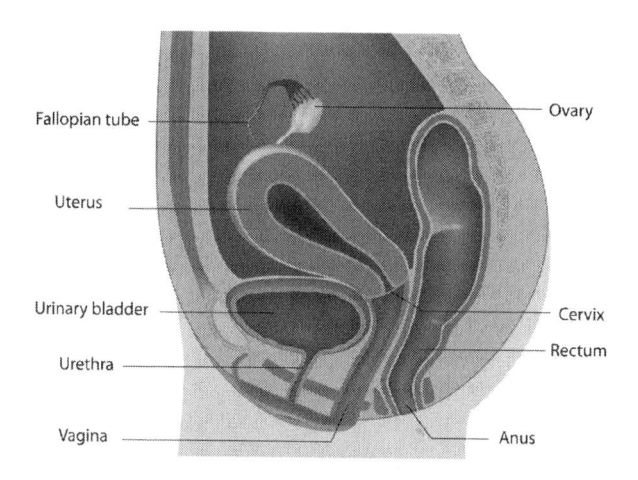

**Fig 4**: Female Reproductive System
(Sagittal View)

# CHAPTER 1.4

## Female Reproductive System

The female reproductive system is mainly made up of the cervix, fallopian tubes, ovaries, uterus and vagina. Its main function is to produce the ovum, an egg, to be fertilized by a sperm. Once the egg is fertilized, it will follow a pathway through the fallopian tube. Upon reaching the uterus, the fertilized egg implants itself to the wall of the uterus where the process of pregnancy will begin. The female reproductive system is also responsible for producing the hormones essential in maintaining the reproductive cycle. The details of the each part of the reproductive system and its functions will be explained below.

### Reproductive Organs

**Fallopian Tubes:** These are hollow connective tubes leading from the ovaries to the uterus. The diameter of the fallopian tube is as thin as a single strand of hair and 10 cm in length. It takes approximately a week for an egg to travel from the ovaries, through the fallopian tubes, to reach the uterus. This is where fertilization usually occurs.

**Ovaries:** These oval-shaped glands lie on both sides of the uterus, varying in shapes and sizes during their lifetime, as well as during the menstrual cycle, from an almond to a walnut shape. They are held in place by ligaments that are attached to the lumbar spine by a muscle called psoas muscles.

**Uterus:** This pear-shaped organ, located centrally in the pelvis, is where the fertilized egg is implanted, which then develops into a baby. The uterus is suspended by ligaments and connective tissue, which is supported by the pelvic floor muscles. The fundus, which is the top of the uterus, lies right above the bladder and the cervix lay, slightly backwards towards the colon. When not menstruating, the uterus normally weighs about 60 grams; its size and weight doubles during menstruation.

The uterus has a variety of natural positions. The most common position is anteverted followed by retroverted. Less common variations includes retroflexed and anteflexed positions. Regardless of the position of the uterus prior to conception, the uterus will assume its natural anteverted position during pregnancy.

The variation in the uterine position is not directly linked to infertility; however, since an anteverted uterus is the most natural position, other positions of the uterus have a higher chance of developing an abnormality that may indirectly contribute to infertility. For example, the naturally occurring retroverted uterus may not have been reported to directly cause infertility; however, it may contribute to symptoms of lower back pain during sexual intercourse or menses. Another possibility is the retroversion of the uterus may be caused by diseases, such as pelvic inflammation diseases (PID), fibroid, surgery due to childbirth, endometriosis, or pelvic adhesion, where it may require a medical intervention, such as surgery, physiotherapy, massage or exercise.

**Vagina:** Vagina is a canal that joins the external part of the opening of this organ to the uterus via the cervix. It is also known as the birth canal that lies anteriorly to the rectum and posterior to the urethra.

Fertility Massage for Women

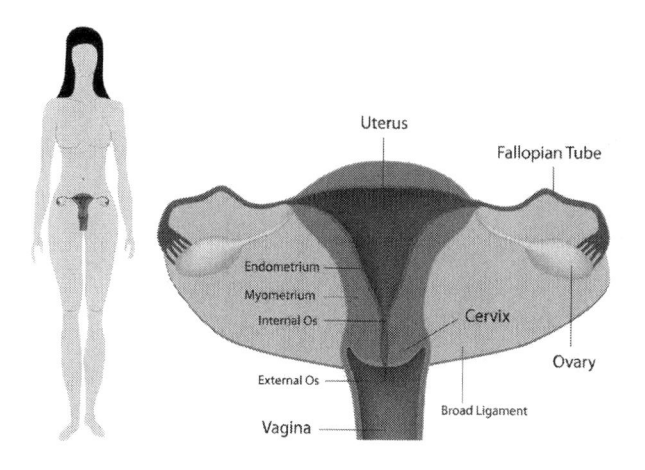

**Fig 5**: Female Reproductive System (Anterior View)

## Ligaments

**Broad Ligament:** The broad ligament is a huge, flat, wide, fold-sheet of peritoneum that is associated with covering the whole surface area of the uterus, fallopian tubes, and ovaries to the pelvic walls. Extending from both sides of the pelvic walls, it serves as a mesentery for these structures to hold it in place, covering the entire anterior and posterior surfaces.

**Ovarian Ligament:** The ovarian ligament is located just below the fallopian tubes. It is a fibrous band of tissues connecting the ovary to the side of the uterus.

**Round Ligament:** A round ligament is responsible for maintaining the uterus in position, especially the anteverted position during pregnancy. Originating from the uterine horn, the part where the uterus meets the fallopian tube, it is connected all the way to the external portion of the vagina by passing through the pelvic area at the inguinal canal. The common stretching pain on the abdomen that is experienced during pregnancy as the uterus expands is associated with this ligament.

**Suspensory Ligament:** The suspensory ligament is attached to the ovary by extending outwards from the ovary to the abdominal wall. Some sources consider this part of the broad ligament, as it does not support any anatomical structure. It functions to contain the ovarian artery and vein, lymphatic system, as well as ovarian nerves.

**Uterosacral Ligament:** The uterosacral ligament is the main ligament responsible for supporting the uterus. Also known as recto-uterine ligament or sacrocervical ligament, these bilateral fibrous bands of tissues are attached from the cervix to the sacrum.

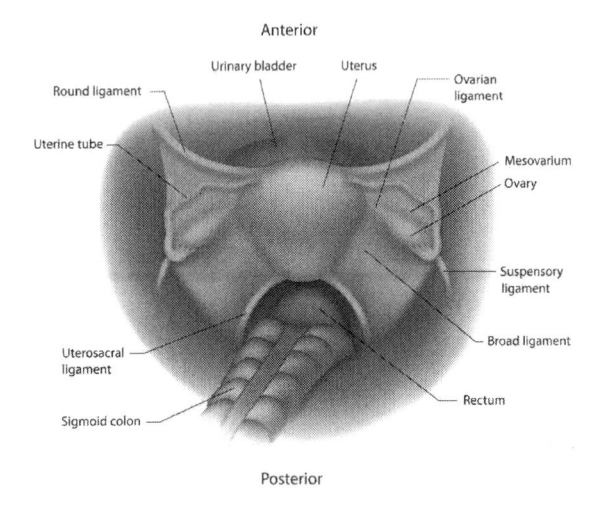

**Fig 6**: Ligaments in Female Reproductive System (Superior View)

## Hormones

**Follicle Stimulating Hormones (FSH):** As the name suggests, the duty of FSH is to stimulate the development of new follicles in the ovary to mature into ovulated eggs. This then leads to the stimulation the production of estrogen. This is the follicular phase of the menstrual cycle where an increase in FSH will further develop only one dominant follicle into one matured ovulated egg.

**Luteinizing Hormones (LH):** LH serves as a signal for ovulation. During the LH surge, the concentration of this hormone increases by up to 10 times the usual amount. Within nine hours, this sudden surge will cause the release of the matured egg from either side of the ovaries. This normally occurs in the middle of the menstruation cycle where fertilization has to occur within one to two days after the release. If no fertilization occurs, the egg begins to disintegrate, along with the inner lining of the uterus, as part of the monthly menstruation cycle.

**Estrogen:** Estrogen is a hormone secreted by the ovaries that helps stop FSH from continuing production, so only one egg will mature in the cycle. The estrogen will then stimulate the pituitary gland to release LH.

**Progesterone:** Progesterone is a hormone also secreted by the ovaries. This hormone is responsible for maintaining the lining of the uterus during the menstrual cycle and through pregnancy.

# CHAPTER 1.5

## Menstrual Cycle

Now that you understand the different parts of the female organs and ligaments, as well as the functions involved in the reproductive system, you will be able to visualize how your menstrual cycle works. This will help you understand how to identify, predict and chart both your menstruation and ovulation period. If you are able to do this accurately, you can delineate the precise fertile period, which increases your chances of successful fertilization following sexual intercourse at the right time, as well as identify a good time for fertility massage.

There are basically two interdependent cycles that occur: i) ovarian cycle; and ii) uterine cycle. The explanation below, of these two cycles, is based on a 28-day cycle.

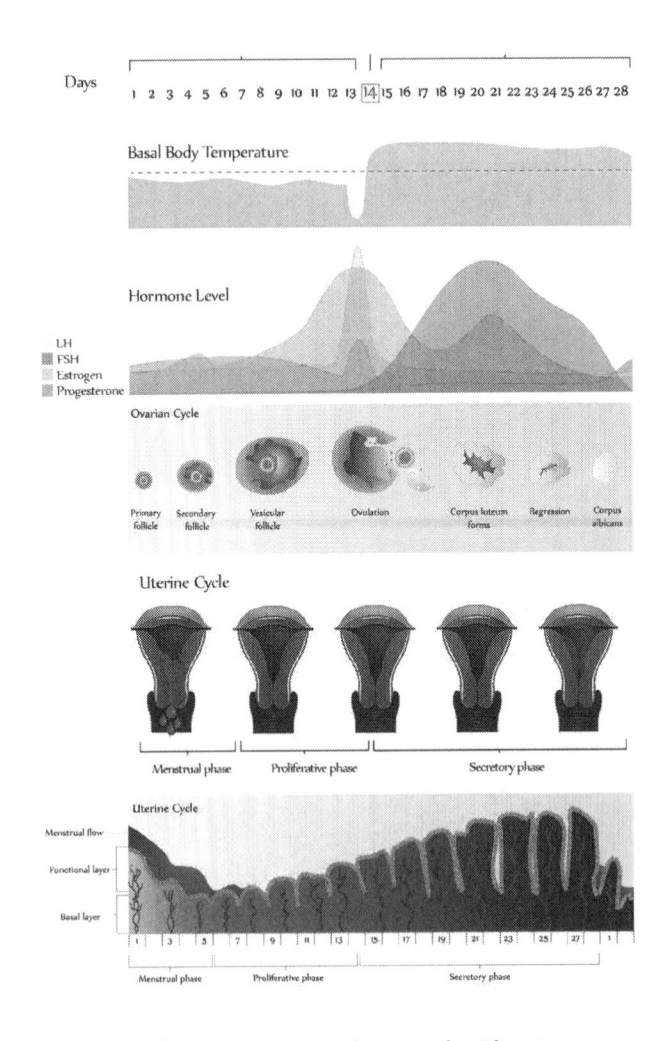

**Fig 7**: Menstruation Cycle Chart

## **Ovarian Cycle**

### Follicular Phase:

- Day 1

- The start of menstruation is also the follicular phase.

- FSH & LH are released into the bloodstream and travel to your ovaries.

- Upon reaching the ovaries, FSH triggers 15-20 eggs to mature in the ovaries, which are now called follicles.

- At the same time, FSH & LH causes the production of estrogen to increase.

- Once the estrogen level is high, it automatically stops the production of the FSH hormones.

- This in turn stops more eggs from maturing — a necessary balance.

- In a few days, only one follicle will become dominant and continues to grow and mature, causing the rest to cease and be reabsorbed back into the body.

- That particular dominant follicle will maintain the production of estrogen.

- The start of endometrial thickening takes place where there is a two to three-fold increase (repair and proliferation).

- There is a continuous growth of the epithelium surface, covering the endometrium where the glands increase in length and number, and spiral arteries elongate, but do not reach the surface.

## Ovulatory Phase:

- About Day 14

- Ovulation occurs, which usually starts midpoint of the menstrual cycle.

- Estrogen will keep rising. Once it reaches its threshold, the release of an LH surge from the brain, causes the dominant follicle to be released from the ovary.

- The matured egg is released from the ovary and starts traveling down the fallopian tubes.

- This phase also causes the increase in quantity and thickening of the mucus in the cervix. The mucus prepares the body for the capture of the sperm, and nourishes the sperm to improve its mobility to increase the chances of the sperm reaching the egg successfully for fertilization to occur.

## Luteal Phase:

- The luteal phase starts immediately after ovulation.

- As the matured egg travels through the fallopian tube, the empty shell left behind in the ovary, called corpus luteum, maintains the secretion of estrogen and progesterone.

- The endometrium will continue thickening in preparation for the implantation of the fertilized egg to the uterus.

- If the sperm successfully fertilizes the egg at this point, conception occurs. The fertilized egg will then continue to travel through the fallopian tube and implant itself onto the uterus. The uterus, already thickened with blood, is ready for the nourishment of the fertilized egg in preparation of pregnancy.

- If no fertilization takes place, the unfertilized egg will pass through the uterus, where the uterus lining breaks down and the next menstrual cycle begins.

# Uterine Cycle

### Menstrual Phase:

- Day 1 - Day 6 (usually lasting three to six days)
- Day 1 is the start of the bleeding phase, where the uterine layer breaks down.
- This menstrual discharge contains old blood, dead endometrial cells, cervical mucus and necrotic tissue.

### Proliferative Phase:

- Day 7 - Day 14
- Once the menstruation ceases, the endometrium layer of the uterus is now at a resting stage and prepares to repair itself.
- Once signaled, the endometrial cells will begin to proliferate again and increase in size, as well as thickness, causing new blood vessels to grow. This is controlled by estrogen.

### Secretary Phase

- Day 16 - Day 28
- Corpus luteum that is producing the progesterone at this time, will trigger the endometrium to start its thickening process in the endometrium cavity of the uterus.

## Fertility Massage for Women

- This secretion of glycogen, fructose and glucose supplies nutrition to the fertilized egg that reaches the uterus.

- If fertilization occurs, the fertilized egg will implant itself in the endometrium.

- If no fertilization takes place, the endometrium will start to degenerate the endometrial lining and be excreted as menstrual blood.

- If there is a delay in the menstrual phase, it is usually due to a delay in the ovulation.

# PART II

# HISTORY & DEVELOPMENT OF MASSAGE & FERTILITY AROUND THE WORLD

# CHAPTER 2.1

## Massage in Traditional Medicine

In many parts of the world, traditional medicine has been a long withstanding healthcare solution and practice before the development and spread of modern western medicine. These traditional medicine practices, in their own unique ways, demonstrate the knowledge and skills of the indigenous people in treating or preventing illnesses; thus, reflecting their wisdom and experience in understanding the nature of human body and its illnesses.

In many studies on traditional medicine, an illness is not necessarily categorized as a physical dysfunction of bodily parts, but originates from an imbalance or disturbance of a person's physical, mental and emotional well-being. Depending on the specific culture and area where traditional medicine is practiced, illnesses, as well as treatments involved, are usually subjected to a sociocultural environment, nature, spiritual world, the cosmos, universe and divine principles. Thus, traditional healing methods, as compared to western medicine, can be considered a more complex means of addressing such conditions as it involves the somatic, emotional, and mental values, as well as mythological based social and ethnic regulative[27].

Although traditional medicine varies from country to country, or region to region, one common form of treatment is always massage. The history of massage is as old as men itself. There is evidence of massage occurring during different periods of prehistoric times, which is scattered all over the world in different nations and cultures. One of the oldest evidence of massage was found to be dated around 3000 B.C in the Chinese written scriptures, called *kong fu*, translating to "mechanical massage". In 1800 B.C, as recorded in the Veda books of wisdom, the Yoga cult in India used respiratory exercises for religious and healing purposes. Egyptian, Persian, as well as Japanese medical literature is full of references to bath

---

[27] Gerber R. & Williams M. (2002). *Geography, Culture, and Education*. Dordrecht, Kluwer Academic Publishers.

Fertility Massage for Women

massages of various kinds[28].

There is also evidence of mechano-therapy for the ancient Phoenicians in Persia, which has been preserved well. Even the ancient Greeks, Herodikos and Hippocrates left behind prescriptions for massage and exercises. Another clear evidence can be found in Pergamon Museum in Berlin, where it displays a 2000 year old artifact, an alabaster relief from the palace of the Assyrian potentate, San Herib, that potrays a clear imagery of massage as realistically as seen in practice today[29].

The purpose of massage is to bring about any of the attributes related to physiological, mechanical, or psychological effects. Through the use of massage, relaxation, relief from pain, reduction of certain types of edema, and an increased range of motion can all be accomplished. Massage is usually combined with other therapeutic measures where massage often provides a form of passive exercise when stretching techniques are used.

As with the case of infertility, massage is a common treatment used in many different cultures and

---

[28] Calver, R. (2002). *The history of massage: An illustrated survey from around the world.* Vermont: Healings Arts Press.

[29] Braun, M., & Simonson, S. (2005). *Introduction to massage therapy.* Philadelphia: Lippincott Williams & Wilkins.

civilizations. This massage treatment is normally coupled with other forms of traditional and ritualistic practices. As mentioned earlier, massage and accompanying treatments not only address the physical causes of infertility, but also the mental, emotional and spiritual needs of the person. This is why many of these treatments also incorporate chanting and mantras during the massage treatments, which more often than not, are connected to spiritual beliefs.

The reason for such a spiritual or religious component in the rituals has to do with the connection of the mental to the emotional state of the body. External issues, such as stress, emotional instability and mental-related issues may affect fertility directly or indirectly; therefore, it is necessary to address the root of these issues. If these areas are not addressed, it may cause the dysfunction of the physical or physiological functions of the body, with the understanding that there is always the issue of safety when using traditional medicines. Considering the availability, affordability and accessibility to traditional medicine, the trend of its proper use will continue to rise, especially where it is widely acceptable, trusted by the community and effective. Therefore, World Health Organization (WHO) advocates the preservation of these traditional medicine practices by creating standard guidelines and regulations[30].

The first step is to be able to monitor the safety, efficacy and quality of these traditional practices to ensure they are adhering to the guidelines of international quality standards. Once established, the community practicing traditional medicine can be assured that they are benefitting directly from these sound practices. Not only that, the intellectual property of the indigenous people, with their healthcare regime and heritage, will also be protected. This would promote the upgrading of knowledge and skills of the traditional medicine practitioner, as well as fostering research and development of innovation in these areas.

Although traditional medicine is gaining recognition and acceptability, there is a lack of research and development around it. Commonly categorized as the traditional and complementary, and alternative medicine (TCAM), there is a lack of support and resources for such a research. Large pharmaceutical companies are willing to fund medical trials in order to develop and sell drugs; thus, fewer resources are made available for studies involving TCAM. On the other hand, due to

---

[30] WHO, *WHO Traditional Medicine Strategy: 2014-2023*.

popularity in TCAM, few organizations, such as the National Center for Complimentary and Alternative Medicine (NCAAM) and Mayo Clinic were established to make research available for the public, by publishing medical journals.

The is also the issue that doctors who are trained in western medical schools have little comprehensive skills, training, or understanding in the field of TCAM, meaning they are unable to give proper recommendations to patients or address the inquiries about TCAM. As with the increase in scientific evidences for TCAM, many doctors are slowly gaining confidence in accepting or recommending it to patients.

Research has been done showing that up to 40% of adults are already, or willing to engage in TCAM, which reflects the steady increasing trend of its popularity[31]. With many medical institutions or organizations combining them with mainstream medicine, there is a new collaboration coined as "integrative medicine". For

---

[31] National Center for Complementary and Alternative Medicine. (2008) Complementary, alternative, or integrative health: What's in a name?. *National Center for Complementary and Integrative Health*, Publication D347. Retrieve from:
https://nccih.nih.gov/sites/nccam.nih.gov/files/CAM_Basics_What_Are_CAIHA_07-15-2014.2.pdf

instance, when medical intervention is not an option for a medically fit patient who is unable to conceive, more and more people turn to TCAM for solutions. At the point of writing this book, there are currently not many research projects already established to demonstrate the effectiveness of massage to address infertility. I believe in due time, if more research is done to prove its effectiveness, massage will be part of the mainstream fertility treatment option.

# CHAPTER 2.2

## China

### Traditional Chinese Medicine (TCM) - Acupressure/Tui Na

The general framework of Traditional Chinese Medicine (TCM) is based on the concept that there is a need for a harmonious environment in a healthy body. The human body is regulated by the life flow of energy, called *qi*. A good flow of energy is essential for good health; thus, the disruption or interruption of this flow will result in an onset of illnesses. With regard to fertility, one of the more commonly used terms is "cold uterus" where there is said to be not enough vital energy flowing through it, which may be the cause of infertility.

There are many ways of correcting this issue, according to TCM, by using Chinese herbalism, acupuncture, acupressure, *tui na*, moxibustion, cupping, *tai qi* and *qi gong*. By deploying these different techniques, the objective is to restore the harmony of one's body by correcting these imbalances in the flow of *qi*. In order to allow the *qi* to flow uninterrupted through the meridian system in the body, the specific points of the body, called acupoints, need to be stimulated when there is a blockage.

Acupuncture is the use of needles to stimulate these points, whereas acupressure aims to achieve the same result by applying physical pressure. *Tui na* can be considered as massaging acts of brushing, kneading, rolling, pressing and rubbing. It deploys a range of motions and movements to stimulate the different acupoints in attempts to unblock the qi and get the energy flowing in the meridians; therefore, all the blockages that are causing infertility may be unlocked with this method. Additionally, the specific acupoints that are associated with improving fertility are stimulated as well.

Incorporating the stimulation on the specific acupoints along the meridian during body massage is done to improve fertility of the body, especially when the massage is done on the lower abdomen. Various movements and motions, including pressing and applying pressure with firm fingertips, not only stimulates the internal organs, but also the relevant acupoints. This causes an increase in blood flow and lymphatic fluid into the pelvic region, loosening the ligaments, muscles, and fascia to allow free movements of the organ from any impending veins or arteries, in order to receive nourishment and oxygen, as well as promote the removal of waste. All this, in turn, would remove any blockages associated with the reproductive system, as well as any barriers that prevent pregnancy.

In recent years, TCM has become very popular around the world with many countries recognizing this practice, including acupuncture and acupressure; thus, requiring the practitioners to abide by specific laws. Some governments enacted laws to regulate TCM practice. Countries like Hong Kong, Malaysia, Australia, Singapore, and most states in United States, have existing regulations stipulated by either Traditional, Complementary or Alternative Medicine Council, Chinese Medicine Board or any equivalent statutory board that comply with TCM Practitioners Act. Hence, practitioners need to be licensed by accredited schools in order to practice either acupuncture or acupressure[32].

Although the practice of acupuncture and acupressure may be accepted in many countries,

---

[32] Ministry of Science and Technology People's Republic of China. (2015). International Traditional Chinese Medicine Program For Cooperation In Science And Technology. *Ministry of Science and Technology of the People's Republic of China.* Retrieve from: http://www.most.gov.cn/eng/policies/regulations/200608/t200608 23_35603.htm.

regarding its ability and effectiveness to treat diseases, criticism still exists. There have been no anatomical, or even histological evidence, of the existence of meridian points based on western medicine. As much as TCM is subjected to scientific research, both in its basis and therapeutic effectiveness, this does not dissuade the followers or believers of TCM from depending on these long standing traditions to help them with their ailments, especially fertility.

## Chinese Taoist Medicine - Chi Nei Tsang

*Chi nei tsang* is a Chinese Taoist tradition practiced by the monks, which means "working on the energy of the internal organ," coming under the branch of *qi gong*, *chi nei tsang* dwells more on the emphasis of the causes of these blockages of energy. Such an energy blockage, derived from suppressed and negative emotions, is deposited in the internal organs. Emotions may include anger, anxiety, depression and fear, as well as stressors such as trauma, improper digestion, bad posture, and drug use, to name a few.

According to traditions, these monks wanted their health to be at its most optimal level, described as a perfectly good healthy body, where they can increase the quality of the life force, *qi*, in order to attain a higher level of spiritual enlightenment. This practice has been almost completely wiped out of existence and only been recently brought back under TCAM.

*Chi nei tsang* has its massages done over the organs in the upper abdomen with deep, soft and gentle movements over the stomach, liver, kidney and parts of the lungs and heart. On the lower abdomen, the massage is performed directly over the reproductive organ to "open up" the organ and release any stress and tension that may be causing blockages due to stored negative emotions, resulting in an improved blood circulation; thus, recreating a healthy reproductive environment in the body and improved fertility.

Aside from the onsite massage of the reproductive organ when performed on women, *chi nei tsang* also regulates women's menstrual cycle and alleviates any premenstrual syndromes, such as diarrhea, constipation, painful cramps, mood swings, depression, etc. This is because the massage on the abdomen helps to release the suppressed emotional charges that linger in the digestive, respiratory, cardiovascular, lymphatic, nervous, endocrine, urinary, reproductive, muscular-skeletal systems, and of course the *qi*.

Considering *chi nei tsang*, is a newly revived tradition, it has not gained as much publicity or popularity as TCM, which has gained a steady foothold in society for its treatment of diseases and ailments over the past years. It can still, however, be found sparsely around the world with more concentration in Southeast Asian countries.

# CHAPTER 2.3

## Malay Archipelago (Southeast Asia)

### Malaysia/Singapore/Brunei - Urut

The indigenous people of Malaysia, Brunei and Singapore have been proactively practicing their own health and beauty regimes for hundreds of years as documented in several manuscripts. Midwifery is amongst one of the most explored disciplines with detailed documentation of pregnancy care, postnatal care, infant care, management of infertility, treatment of ailments, nutritional advice, and the use of herbs and spices as medicine.

*Urut*, which means massage in the Malay language, is a huge subject area for the Malay culture. The Malays use therapeutic massage to treat different ailments for different reasons and purposes. They have prenatal massage, postnatal massage, infant massage, fertility massage (for both men and women), and treatments for ailments including soreness, sprains, strains, nerves or muscular problems.

With regards to fertility for men, *urut batin* (manhood massage), has a wide range of treatment regimes to address ailments, such as erectile dysfunction, low sperm quality or count, prostate issues or premature ejaculation. Women on the other hand, also have a set of massage regimes, *sengkak*, that is specially performed on women with infertility issues, who have already given birth have a prolapse uterus, painful menstruation cramps, irritable bowel or painful intercourse, amongst other reasons. Massage may be used with the combination of topical or ingested herbs, alongside other practices such as *ganggang, tungku* and *tuam*.

*Ganggang*, which can be described as a treatment in the form of vaginal steaming, is part of the Malay traditional medicine for women. It involves a procedure where a woman sits on a specially crafted wooden stool that is hollowed in the center, exposing the external vaginal area. A bowl of aromatic herbs is then placed on the ground, between her legs under the chair and heated up. The steam, or smoke, is directed to waft up the confined space of the stool to reach the exposed vaginal area. The alternative, simpler method is by wearing a sarong, standing with legs apart, and heated aromatic herbs placed between the legs.

## Fertility Massage for Women

*Ganggang*, is beneficial in reducing lochia and excessive vaginal discharge and mucus, as well as eliminate bacteria that cause unpleasant smells and irritation. Although *ganggang* is part of the health routine and beauty regime for women, it is highly recommended for women who are trying to conceive, and for recovering postnatal women who went through vaginal delivery. According to tradition, this practice indirectly expedites the tightening of the vagina.

Another traditional treatment to optimize the health of the uterus includes a hot compress, called *tungku* or *tuam*, depending on the shape and type of material used as the tool. It consists of either a flat stone or short iron rod that is preheated and wrapped with fresh leaves and herbs, followed by layers of cloth. This heat compression is best done routinely, following delivery, following a miscarriage, or even during menstruation. The compression is directly pressed over the uterus to aid in the release of toxins, expulsion of wind, and breaking down of blood clots. This helps to clear the uterus of dead skin cells, or necrotic tissues, and reduce scarring and adhesion, which is necessary for a successful conception and healthy pregnancy.

The status of Malay traditional medicine practices has gained popularity in recent years. What was once thought to be a superstitious or backward practice, is now receiving a lot of attention in recent times with the progression of science and technology. Many independent research documents explain how and why specific practices are effective. For example, new findings in the botanical compounds used in medicinal herbs promote the popularity and acceptance of such practices.

A research done by World Health Organization (WHO) surveying postnatal women all over the world has shown that Malaysia has had the lowest postnatal depression rate in the world [33]. WHO promotes the traditional medicinal practices in countries like Malaysia, of which the low rate of postnatal depression has been associated with the prevalent practice of Malay traditional postnatal care [34]. With such acknowledgement of the effectiveness of Malay massages in postnatal care, more research has been encouraged to promote the use of Malay traditional medicine and practices.

This too has extended the use of massage and other safe traditional practices for infertility, which is gaining acceptance and popularity in a multicultural landscape in

---

[33] Oates, M., Cox, J., Neema, S., Asten, P., Glangeaud-Freudenthal, N., Figueiredo, B., & Gorman, L. et al. (2004). Postnatal depression across countries and cultures: A qualitative study. The British Journal of Psychiatry, 184(46), s10-s16.

[34] Kit, L., Kick, G., & Ravindran, J. (1997). Incidence of postnatal depression in Malaysian women. Journal of Obstetrics and Gynaecology Research, 23(1), 85-89.

Southeast Asia. With its acceptance, more people are becoming more open to this regime and have come to seek this uterus massage, *sengkak*, as a means to improve their fertility.

## Indonesia - Pijat

Malays from Indonesia, and Malays from Singapore, Malaysia and Brunei, have many overlapping practices in their health and beauty regimes, considering how they share similar ancestral lineage and heritage. In treating infertility issues, Indonesian tradition practices *pijat*, massage, as well as the use of *jamu*, medicine. *Pijat* has many similarities to the Malay massage, *urut*, whereas *jamu* uses herbs from roots, tree barks, leaves, flowers, fruits, nuts and seeds, to create a concoction either for consumption or external application. This promotes health and wellness, and prevents and cures ailments.

Used in conjunction with each other, *jamu* and *pijat* are known to cure infertility problems for both men and women. Specific *jamu* concoctions can be made for specific ailments, including increasing libido, improving sperm quality or quantity for men, and addressing specific menstrual issues or hormonal issues for woman.

The basic holistic approach in Indonesian treatment regimes for any illness or ailments involves focusing on three important factors: *jiwa* (mind), *raga* (body), and *sukma* (spirit) in order to achieve optimum health. Accordingly, there is a need to address all the factors concurrently, and if any of these three factors is not addressed, then there will be no success in the treatments.

The three main components of treatment, in order to have optimum health, include: i) allowing the mind (*jiwa*) to stay calm, relaxed, and positive; ii) detoxifying the body (*raga*) with jamu to maintain stamina and good looks with positive energy and appearance; and iii) improving the *sukma*, or spiritual life, to enhance willpower, energy and spirited life. Similar to the Malay culture, besides massage and the use of *jamu*, there are many practices that makeup the infertility treatment including *ratus*, similar to *ganggang* (feminine vaginal steam) and *mandian* (herbal bath).

# CHAPTER 2.4

## Latin America

### Mexico - Mayan Abdominal Massage

The Mayan civilization is very steeped in their knowledge of traditional medicine, following centuries of oral traditions passed down from generations of shamanic healers. Their traditional healing method includes various practices, such as herbal medicine, spiritual baths, chanting practices and spiritual healing.

The abdominal massage technique is used to treat various abdominal illnesses including massaging displaced organs back to its actual location. Thus making this abdominal massage indirectly effective in improving fertility. According to tradition, a misplaced uterus may impact neighboring organs, especially the colon and bladder, which on top of causing pain, can complicate conception. In addition, a displaced uterus can increase susceptibility to cramps, painful intercourse and the growth of uterine fibroids or polyps.

Using deep tissue massage, the slow massage action gently restores the uterus to its original location, increases internal balance, as well as homeostasis within the pelvic area. This also alleviates the pressure on the surrounding organs, including the arteries and veins, as well as the lymph nodes that may be caused by the displaced uterus. Once all is in order and in balance, the uterus will be in place and there will be better blood circulation; thus, pregnancy can occur more easily.

Mayan abdominal therapy was made popular by Dr. Arvigo, an American-born citizen who was an apprentice of the last descendant of Mayan civilization, of a shamanic healer, Don Elijio, in Belize, Mexico. Dr. Arvigo developed and documented the abdominal massage technique under the title: Arvigo Technique Mayan Abdominal Therapy (ATMAT). Dr. Arvigo took these ancient methods of abdominal massage, and with a modern approach, consolidated the techniques and supported them with evidence in order to make the therapy widely accepted in modern society.

# CHAPTER 2.5

## Japan

### Reiki

Originating from a Japanese Buddhist, Reiki is a self-healing method that uses the transference of universal energy, as the Japanese call *ki*, through the palms of one's hands to aid in healing one or others. Traditional Japanese Reiki involves placing the palms over different parts of the body without any contact, in order to transfer energy using intuitive sense. Western Reiki, however, uses a systematic hand placement, with skin contact on the body for this transference of energy. Western Reiki may arguably be considered massage as it has a component of touch. Although it is not vigorous in any way, it still is considered a basic form of massage.

Reiki is not a manipulation of soft tissues, organs or muscles. Reiki boosts fertility by providing emotional and mental balance to help women with fertility. The inability to conceive creates a negative field surrounding a woman, which blocks her ki, which in turn creates a more hostile environment for conception. The aim of Reiki is to restore a woman's energy field in order to clear, repair and unblock her energy field by bringing equilibrium to her mind and body.

# CHAPTER 2.6

## Worldwide

### Massage Therapy in Physiotherapy / Physical Therapy

Physiotherapy, also known as Physical Therapy, is an allied healthcare profession that aims to treat individuals with conditions that limit their mobility functions. This form of therapy is customized according to the individual, using treatments to improve mobility, reduce pain, restore function, prevent disability and improve overall quality of life. Physiotherapists, or physical therapists, provide care for people from newborns to the elderly in various disposition, including hospitals, private clinics, schools, sports and fitness facilities, nursing homes and health agencies.

Originating all the way back to the times of Hippocrates in 460 BC, many physicians were known to have practiced some form of physical therapy in terms of massage, manual therapy, and hydrotherapy to treat people with various conditions. The earliest documentation of physical therapy was by Per Henrik Ling in 1813, where he developed the first Professional group called the Royal Central Institute of Gymnastics of which many other countries subsequently followed, forming related institues of massage and medical gymnastics[35].

With the progression of physical therapy, nurses in the 19th century were trained in physical education including massage and remedial exercise as aftercare for patients after orthopedic surgeries. Shortly after 1921, there was a research group in the physical therapy movement who started publishing medical research journals on the effectiveness of physical therapy. Ever since then, International Physical Therapist Confederations were created around the world. The organization plays a significant role in promoting the advancement of this form of therapy around the world.

By using a wide range of accepted theoretical, as well as scientifically explained clinical applications, physiotherapist/physical therapists are capable of restoring, maintaining, and also promoting the optimal

---

[35] Beck, *Theory & Practice Of Therapeutic Massage*

physical form and function of their clients. These therapists would be involved in the diagnosis process, management of the dysfunctions in the client's movements, and enhancement in the limitation of physical disabilities to achieve the optimal fitness level and well-being for an improved quality of life.

Recently in the United States, few physical therapist is attempting to address fertility related issues in women using massage in their independent clinics. One such attempt is by Jennifer Mercier where she developed the Mercier Technique. The manual physical manipulation, i.e., massage, is noted to enhance female well-being and restore the physiologic functions and anatomic structures of the female pelvis. It is a mild, non-invasive technique, which is also designed to help women reconnect with their emotional and spiritual selves, and ultimately restore inner health and balance.

According to Mercier, women who suffer from chronic pain due to conditions such as dyspareunia, endometriosis, dysmenorrhea, etc., can be severely debilitated to the point that it could lead to impairment of the reproductive function. The pain may originate anywhere from any pelvic organ, be it the bladder, uterus, fallopian tubes, the ovaries, etc. Majority of such conditions are caused by surgeries or chronic inflammation, e.g., pelvic inflammatory disease.

Mercier reported that those who have undergone such therapy have reported improved physical and psychological well-being, with concurrent improvement in their quality of life. Although only one peer review study has been conducted to validate the benefits of her technique, a number of testimonials have been collected, with reports of relief from chronic pelvic pain, dyspareunia, and dysmenorrhea, as well as restoration of female fertility after undergoing the Mercier Technique.

Another physical therapist, Belinda Wurn, also developed her own technique for abdominal massage therapy, which was further developed to help women with infertility issues. During the 1980s, Belinda Wurn underwent chemotherapy and radiation after being diagnosed with cervical cancer. This caused the scars in her pelvic structures to adhere to one another, leading to a condition called "frozen pelvis". Due to the lack of any tangible progress with modern medicine, Belinda resorted to alternative methods of therapy.

In her search, she developed a non-invasive manual physical therapy, naming it the "Wurn Technique". It is used to mobilize fibrotic structures. Currently, the Wurn Technique has massage techniques allowing strategic manipulation of internal structures and loosening of abdomino-pelvic adhesions.

At the start, this new treatment modality was only backed primarily by outcomes, i.e., increased pregnancy rates after the therapy. Refusing to be overcome by the lack of available literature supporting her technique, Wurn later explored the physiologic and anatomic nature of adhesions and constructed a new theory that would substantiate her practice. A few studies have shown that manual manipulation disrupts the integrity of connective tissues, which is the primary component of adhesions. This study further found that manual manipulation, i.e., massage, breaks down connective tissues and loosens fibrotic structures. Thereafter, a number of scientific explorations have been conducted to further prove the efficacy of this noninvasive and strategically applied manual manipulation of pelvic structures[36].

Just as how sweaters can be taken apart thread by thread, the Wurn Technique claims to tear down adhesions, cross-link after cross-link. Several peer-reviewed journals highlighted the technique's ability to relieve pain and promote soft tissue mobility without placing the patient at a higher risk for adhesions; in contrast to more invasive forms of adhesiolysis, such as surgery or medication. The technique was also found to be effective in reopening previously blocked fallopian tubes, which improves IUI and IVF success rates[37]. In

---

[36] Wurn, B., Wurn, L., Roscow, A., King, R., Heuer, M., & et al. (2008). Treating fallopian tube occlusion with a manual pelvic physical therapy, *Alternative Therapies, 14*(1), 18-23.

[37] Wurn et al., *Treating female infertility and improving IVF pregnancy rates with a manual physical therapy technique.*

the Journal of Clinical Medicine, the Wurn Technique was also useful in treating bowel obstructions caused by adhesions[38].

Currently, the Wurn Technique is practiced only in United States. Despite the insufficient number of studies conducted to evaluate the benefits of the Wurn Technique, there is potential for future research in the field of female reproductive issues.

## Others

Another treatment that is found in Europe, is the Abdominal Sacral Technique developed by alternative medicine experts stating that emotional and neurologic activity is centered in the abdomen. It argues that disregarding this important area, means neglecting the body's deepest tension. Especially that the abdomen is supplied by the same neural connections as those that connect to organs, muscles and connective tissues; therefore, if any part of the body, for example an organ or a muscle, is obstructed, misaligned, or malfunctioned in some way, the rest of the body would be dysfunctional.

---

[38] Rice, A. D. (2013). Manual physical therapy for non-surgical treatment of adhesion-related small bowel obstructions: Two case reports., J. Clin. Med, 2(1), 1-12.

## Fertility Massage for Women

The body's immune system is concentrated within the abdominal cavity and is closely linked to functions of the female reproductive system. As such, obstructions or disrupted abdominal cavity functions could lead to an impairment of female fertility.

The abdominal sacral massage, is described as a deep massage that is both mild and non-invasive. This technique is based on its ability to realign abdominal structures, release tension and increase abdominal muscle strength. It also improves the flow of blood, lymph and neural signals. Further, toxins are released from the body, while nutrients are better absorbed.

Abdominal pelvic massage attempts to relieve abdomino-pelvic obstructions and realign structures to enhance neural connections, subsequently improving female reproductive functions. In fact, recipients of this alternative treatment have reported relief from chronic pelvic pain, improved sleep and reduced levels of stress. It is currently practiced only in Europe such as U.K, Scotland and Ireland.

# PART III

DEVELOPMENT OF MALAY UTERUS MASSAGE™ BY SALWA SALIM, UTERUS HEAT THERAPY & VAGINAL STEAM THERAPY

# CHAPTER 3.1

## Malay Midwifery & Women's Reproductive Health

In recent years, there were many attempts to compile and document the Malay traditional medicine practices. Books, such as *Dunia Perbidanan Melayu,* The World of Malay Midwifery, or *Ensiklopedia Perbidanan Melayu,* Encyclopedia of Malay Midwifery, have successfully collated informations to explain in extensive details, topics including: i) anatomy and physiology of the female body; ii) illnesses related to the female reproductive system; iii) history of midwifery, pregnancy and the birth process; iv) prenatal and postnatal care (natural and Caesarian births); v) intensive treatment and the importance of postnatal care for women in the confinement period; vi) nutrition; vii) welcoming a newborn into the world; viii) infant care; ix) illnesses and treatment of newborns; x) miscarriages; xi) infertility, and many more.

These books are examples of the extensive knowledge and experience of all those who are in the field of midwifery. Before modern medical science and technology reached this part of the world, midwifery was an exemplification portraying the Malays' deep understanding of the internal organs, nervous system and skeletal system, as well as the their functions.

The accuracy of their understanding can now be explained by modern medical sciences, which shows wisdom in traditional medicine. Even the equivalent word for "uterus" has up to five different names in the Malay language, *rahim, merian, peranak, peranakan* and *penyawa* — that shows the vastness and the development in their linguistic knowledge of the human anatomy.

Since western medicine has taken prevalence as the primary healthcare for women giving birth, traditional midwives have limited roles, considering the strict regulations imposed on them. Even so, this does not discourage them to carry out the postnatal care practices that are still very much practiced today; however, with the gaining popularity of home-births practiced by many in the modern world that bear a striking resemblance to successful home-births performed by Malay midwives, it would be a matter of time before midwives begin to reclaim their traditional practices and get recognized for it in their own right. Nevertheless, the research done by World Health Organization (WHO) that surveys postnatal women all over the world showed that

## Fertility Massage for Women

Malaysia has the lowest postnatal depression in the world, attributing it to Malay traditional postnatal care practices[39]. This has encouraged not only the research and development of these traditional practices, but also the conviction of many individuals from different multicultural groups of these practices.

Despite the reduction in the number of traditional midwives; midwifery, or massage, has regained a respectful position in the community for its vital contribution to a mother's postnatal care. Postnatal care is a service not provided by medical professionals. It is safe to say that this is still very much alive and accepted region-wide. The *tukang urut* (massage therapist/masseur), can be found in almost every big and small town across Malaysia, Singapore and Indonesia. More often than not, these massage therapists are well equipped with the knowledge and skills to perform traditional massage and other treatments.

---

[39] Oates, M. R et al. *Postnatal Depression Across Countries And Cultures: A Qualitative Study*

# CHAPTER 3.2

## Malay Uterus Massage™ by Salwa Salim, Uterus Heat Therapy & Vaginal Steam Therapy

### Malay Uterus Massage™ by Salwa Salim

There are many techniques in the Malay art of massage that is unique to a certain part of the body for specific purposes. *Sengkak* is a series of movements performed on the lower abdomen directly over the uterus for purposes of menstrual or menopausal related problems, incontinence, postnatal issues, prolapsed uterus, irritable bowel syndrome and painful intercourse amongst other reproductive health issues. *Sengkak* is a unique and sought after massage technique, known even amongst the non-Malays women in the geographical region where it is found as a form of therapeutic massage for women.

Fertility Massage for Women

As for Malay Uterus Massage™ by Salwa Salim, it is created based on this *sengkak* technique in order to standardize and ensure safe practices, as well as deliver quality and effective results. There are two main categories where M.U.M.™ is applicable in cases of infertility:

1) **Professional M.U.M.™ Fertility Massage:** A series of techniques performed by trained therapists as part of massage treatment for women with fertility or reproductive issues. As the name suggests, the technique stems from the Malay traditional practices that has undergone generations of trial and error and reports to be effective. The techniques of M.U.M.™ has been further developed by the Mummy's Fertility team to ensure that it meets the latest requirements and standards of massage and safety of practices. With a deeper knowledge and understanding of modern anatomy and physiology, the effectiveness of this techniques can be correlated to positive outcomes of specific ailments with present day medical insights.

2) **Self M.U.M.™ Fertility Massage:** Designed for individuals to provide aftercare self maintainence on themselves on a regular basis, the techniques are the simplified versions of Professional M.U.M.™ Fertility Massage, which are taught by qualified therapist. It's suitable to be self-performed. Regular

self-massage is vital in maintaining the health of the uterus.

Professional M.U.M™ Fertility Massage is not merely about the physical manual manipulation of the uterus only. It also includes areas in relation to the female reproductive region. In *sengkak* it is specifically done on the lower abdomen only. However our improved techniques involves massaging other related parts, such as around the hips, along the pubic bone, and all the way around the back to the sacrum and lower back and spine. It is crucial that massage is done at these region because of the relationship the reproductive organ has with its surrounding and connections of the major muscles and ligaments that are holding up the uterus in the hollow space of the pelvic bone.

Competent therapists are able to perform M.U.M.™ by first locating the uterus through touch using her fingers and/or hands. She will be able to detect if the uterus is in its original location, prolapsed or tilted to either side of the body. An experienced competent therapist may also discern any notable abnormalities by the size or texture of the uterus or the surrounding organs, as well as identifying if there is tightness or tension in the surrounding ligaments and muscles, leading the uterus to be constricted or tilted. The ability to detect abnormalities is also dependent on many factors, such as the shape and size of the individual. For example, it is easier to identify the uterus within a flat abdomen, compared to one beneath a thick layer of fat.

## Fertility Massage for Women

Nevertheless, M.U.M.™ can be performed on all women.

A healthy uterus is a suspended organ in the pelvic bowl. One of the aim of M.U.M.™ is to loosen all tightness in the muscles and ligaments that may cause the uterus to be displaced, breaking down any adhesions or new buildup of scar tissues, and remove any obstructions that may impede the uterus or the surrounding structures. According to the Malay practice, it is common for women to suffer cases of *"rahim jatuh"* which translates to "fallen uterus" or can be referred to as the early onset of mild prolapsed uterus or displaced/misaligned uterus. The signs and symptoms are very common amongst women who are not aware that they be suffering from this condition (See Chapter 4.2). One of the techniques in M.U.M.™ taking after *sengkak,* involves an *upward* pushing technique to release the uterus from this unnatural position. With regular sessions, the uterus is strengthened so that it is reinstated to be freely suspending again in its natural position. This particular massage technique is not meant to change the natural position of the uterus, for example from a naturally retroverted position to an anteverted position. The technique is mainly to reposition the uterus and ovaries in its supposed natural and original location.

On top of that, part of the technique involves stroking, pressing and rubbing. These aid in the breakdown of scar tissues or adhesions, that may cause any obstructions in the system. Professional M.U.M™ Fertility Massage is best done with Uterus Heat Therapy, which can greatly help in clearing out and cleansing the uterus. These unwanted materials will then be released with the next menstrual cycle. This is notably a great benefit for women who have undergone past pregnancies, miscarriages, abortions or operations.

When both Professional M.U.M™ Fertility Massage and Self M.U.M.™ Fertility Massage techniques are done regularly and continuously, chances of conception will improve. Just like any form of therapy, exercise, or diet regime, M.U.M.™ is not a one-time treatment where the client will miraculously become pregnant after one session. It has to be performed routinely, both professionally and by the individual.

## Uterus Heat Therapy

As part of the Professional M.U.M.™ Fertility Massage sequence, uterus heat therapy is either done concurrently or immediately after M.U.M.™. Similar to *tungku* and *tuam* mentioned in Chapter 2.3, a stone wrapped with selected herbs or herbal ball is used as a heat compression tool. It is pressed down with a stationary rotational movement at multiple focal points over the abdomen, pelvis, sacrum and groin areas. These are the crucial areas where the reproductive system lies, the junctions and attachments of the muscles and ligaments and the location of the lymph nodes respectively.

The use of heat or thermotherapy, is a common treatment used to facilitate massage as it has properties that helps to relieve stiffness and chronic aches. When heat is applied over these areas, the temperature of the tissues will rise which increases blood flow and stimulate circulation in the areas. This will aid in increased speed in releasing toxin and helps the flow of extra nutrients into the area to assist in the recovery and healing process. When directly pressed over the uterus, it helps to breakdown the endometrium layer by dislodging any dead endometrium cells and tissues that are stagnant and still stuck to the uterus walls, including any old stale blood and any dead tissues.

## Vaginal Steam Therapy

Taking after the Malay traditional practice of *ganggang*, vaginal steam therapy is a unique treatment using the healing properties of selected herbs and thermotherapy in the form of heat and steam for the healing and cleansing of the external genital and anal areas. Steam is known to have disinfecting properties to kill germs and bacteria. With the vaginal steam therapy, it is beneficial in disinfecting the vaginal area to keep it clear from bacteria, eliminate any unpleasant smells, irritation or itch, improves expulsion of excess mucus, tighten and strengthen the vagina, and reduce excessive vaginal discharge. The use of the selected herbs infuses its healing properties and eliminate bad odor, leaving the area genital and anal area feeling cleaner, healthy and fresh. The modality of vaginal steam therapy is described in Chapter 2.3.

## Is M.U.M.™ Suitable for Me?

M.U.M.™ is not just for women with infertility issues. It is recommended for all post puberty women as part of their regular health maintenance of their reproductive system. M.U.M.™ is suitable for women in the management of menstrual problems, abdominal discomfort, menopausal symptoms, infertility issues, and postnatal care. It is however more popular amongst women with fertility issues, as it has a track record for resolving women's reproductive health. M.U.M.™ is suitable even for conditions like endometriosis, blocked or twisted fallopian tubes, irregular ovulation, amenorrhea, irregular menstrual cycles leading to lack of ovulation, pelvic adhesions, or idiopathic issues where there are no particular reasons for infertility, which directly or indirectly leads to infertility.

In general, M.U.M.™ is performed in conjunction with a full body massage, hence called: M.U.M.™ Fertility Massage. On top of the direct benefits of massage on the reproductive organs, massage is usually done to relieve stress. Research studies have shown the relationship of massage to stress reduction, as it lowers the stress hormones and cortisol levels in the body. Considering stress is an inhibiting factor to fertility, a full body massage can directly boost your chances of pregnancy.

Fertility Massage for Women

The cautionary measures to take note of when doing M.U.M.™ is that it is prohibited to be performed on women who are pregnant, after implantation of an embryo following IVF, insemination following IUI procedures, immediately after a natural or C section delivery, and on women with any medical conditions or procedures done involving the abdomen or pelvis area. In any case, it is always best to seek a doctor's approval.

The general rule before any massage is to first seek your medical practitioner's approval. Prior to starting the M.U.M.™ treatment, the attending therapist will assess your condition to evaluate if you are a good candidate to receive both Professional M.U.M.™ Fertility Massage and Self M.U.M.™ Fertility Massage, to ensure you have no contraindication to have massage performed on you. If there are no indicators that prevent you from having the massage, you can proceed. Massage, in general, does not have negative side affects if done with care.

## Who is Qualified to Perform Malay Uterus Massage™?

Professional M.U.M.™ Fertility Massage can only be performed by a trained therapist that is certified by Mummy's Fertility Pte. Ltd. (Singapore). The therapist must already possess sound knowledge of anatomy and physiology and skills in performing full body massage. The therapist will need to be able to determine if the individual is a good candidate by assessing their body condition, personal or medical history, menstrual cycle, menstrual symptoms and discuss their infertility history and problems before performing Professional M.U.M.™ Fertility Massage. Each therapist needs to have a particular set of understanding of the female reproductive system and is then required to undergo specialized training to fully understand the requirements and techniques of Professional M.U.M.™ Fertility Massage.

As for Self M.U.M.™ Fertility Massage, it may be done by any individual after attending trainings/workshops/private tutorials by a M.U.M.™ instructor. It is crucial that the individual has the correct tools, skills and guidance prior to performing the massage. Part II of this book, which displays the exact steps of the Self M.U.M.™ Fertility Massage can be obtained through Mummy's Fertility Pte Ltd (Singapore) during sessions with our therapist or through our trainings and workshops.

# CHAPTER 3.3

## Practical Application

### Understanding and Identifying Your Menstrual Cycle

Understanding your menstrual cycle is a crucial part of M.U.M.™ as it defines the exact window period to perform fertility massage. With this, you will also be able to indicate the period not to perform the massage. Once you are familiar with your menstrual cycle, you will be able to plan when to perform M.U.M.™, as well as when is the best time for intercourse.

The menstrual cycle is when a woman's body undergoes natural changes in the sexual reproductive system in different phases, in the ovaries and the uterus. The uterine cycle consists of menstruation, proliferative, and the secretory phase in preparation of the uterus for pregnancy and the ovarian cycle consists of the follicular phase, ovulation, and luteal phase to prepare the egg.

Both cycles are controlled by the endocrine system.

The length of a menstrual cycle varies among women ranging between 21 to 35 days, of which 28 days is the median average of a cycle. Day 1 denotes the first day of your menstruation period and the number continues on until you start your next menstruation period. Under normal circumstances, you will notice a pattern, where the number of menstrual days are consistent. The ideal and healthy menstrual cycle revolves around the same number of days, where you will able to predict your next menstrual period. The best way to identify your menstrual cycle is by charting it on your period calendar, or monthly cycle calendar.

## Identifying Your Ovulation Period and Charting Your Menstrual Cycle

One way of identifying your ovulation period is by charting your basal body temperature. This procedure includes taking your temperature first thing in the morning when you wake, before doing any activities after at least of 5 hours of sleep. The sensitivity of a basal thermometer records even minute changes up to 0.1 degrees. When observing your body basal temperature, your ovulation day falls on the day before you see a sudden spike of 0.2 - 0.4 degrees Celsius in your temperature and it is maintained until your menstruation period. Over time you will see a pattern in your ovulation cycle, and you will be able to understand your body rhythm and plan for sexual intercourse a few days before the expected temperature spike.

Another method that normally accompanies the basal body temperature charting is the charting of your cervical mucus. With all these changes in your body, your cervical mucus will change in terms of its amount, color, texture and viscosity throughout your cycle. When your cervical mucus is dry, sticky, cloudy or creamy, this is an indication that you are not at your fertile period, which occurs before or after your ovulation period. However, when the mucus becomes clear and slippery, most commonly described as that of a raw egg white, it indicates the fertile period. This cervical mucus is part of your body's system to nourish the eggs and help the sperm travel more efficiently to reach fertilization. You can find the resources and extensive description on how to chart your menstrual cycle through our Fertile Body Model™ program.

## The Four Seasonal Phase of the Menstrual Cycle

Women's bodies are very much in sync to nature and the surrounding. Ideally the consistency of menstrual cycle should be like clockwork, just like the lunar cycle of the moon completing its revolution around the earth in 28 days. What is described as mother nature, is very much attune to a women's character of being nurturing and their likeness to giving birth to life. Just like how the four seasons change throughout the year, giving rise to different environments, so does the female body.

The metaphor of the four seasons — autumn, winter, spring and summer — will be used in this part of the book to correspond to the four phases of the menstrual cycle. These seasons relate to changes in the female body. By identifying the different stages your body goes through, you can easily identify at which stage you are in and when it is best to perform M.U.M.™ or have sexual intercourse.

## The Four Seasons of the Menstrual Cycle

### AUTUMN

**Week 1:** Day 1 - Day 6

**Season:** Week of Menses

**Explanation:** Autumn marks the end of the cycle that starts in spring. The cycle is complete, the fruit is harvested, the leaves start to shed, and everything is cleared to make way for a new beginning. Similar to your menstrual phase, this is where the menses begins and lasts normally between 5 - 6 days. The uterus disintegrates the endometrium layer, forming the menstruation blood, by shedding the soft tissue and blood vessels.

**Recommendations:** Not recommended for any forms of massage.

**Table 1:** The Four Seasons of
The Menstrual Cycle (Autumn)

## WINTER

**Week 1:** Day 7 - Day 14

**Season:** Week After Menses

**Explanation:** This is the quiet period of time where, typical of winter, life retreats in preparation for the upcoming spring for the growth of a new life. This is the phase where FSH will stimulate the eggs in the ovaries so that it may start to grow and mature. Once this egg matures, it then secretes progesterone to signal the uterus to prepare the lining of the blood vessels in the endometrium. Otherwise, on the surface, like winter, everything is quiet and calm with not much activity happening.

**Recommendations:** Best time to perform M.U.M.™

**Table 1:** The Four Seasons of The Menstrual Cycle (Winter)

## SPRING

**Week 1:** Day 15 - Day 21

**Season:** Week of Ovulation

**Explanation:** Now comes spring, where life starts to appear and flowers begin to bloom. The matured egg is released in the fallopian tube. The egg, at this point, will start to travel down the fallopian tube waiting to be fertilized. This window period is the most fertile stage in a woman's cycle. This is when the uterine lining thickens in preparation for the arrival of a fertilized egg.

**Recommendations:** M.U.M.™ is recommended right before the ovulation, up to 30 minutes before sexual intercourse to prepare the body for conception. All forms of massage should stop immediately after insemination (naturally or with IUI), as well as after implantation (IVF). M.U.M.™ not to be done if suspected pregnant.

**Table 1: The Four Seasons of The Menstrual Cycle (Spring)**

## SUMMER

**Week 1:** Day 21-Day 28

**Season:** Week Before Menses

**Explanation:** Summer-time is when fruit ripen and the harvest begins. Continuing on the thickening process of the uterus, if the egg is not fertilized by a sperm it will start to disintegrate. If no fertilization takes place, the endometrium will start to degenerate the endometrial lining and be excreted as menstrual blood. This causes the next cycle of menstrual phase to begin.

**Recommendations:** M.U.M.™ is not to be done if pregnancy is suspected. M.U.M.™ is permissible only if you are certain you are not pregnant.

**Table 1**: The Four Seasons of
The Menstrual Cycle (Summer)

## Best Time, Condition & Environment to Perform M.U.M.™

Once you have successfully charted your menstrual cycle, you will be able to identify the best time to perform M.U.M.™. Whether you are doing Professional M.U.M™ Fertility Massage or Self M.U.M.™ Fertility Massage, a certain number of hours need to be satisfied in order to see marked results. Professional M.U.M™ Fertility Massage is usually done with a full body massage, Self M.U.M.™ Fertility Massage is done directly on-site over the abdomen which takes about 10-20 minutes to complete.

| | | | | | | | |
|---|---|---|---|---|---|---|---|
| Week 1 Autumn | 1 💧 | 2 💧 | 3 💧 | 4 💧 | 5 💧 | 6 💧 | 7 |
| Week 2 Winter | 8 | 9 | 10 | 11 | 12 | 13 | 14 🪷 |
| Week 3 Spring | 15 | 16 | 17 | 18 | 19 | 20 | 21 |
| Week 4 Summer | 22 | 23 | 24 | 25 | 26 | 27 | 28 |

**LEGEND**

28 Day Cycle

💧 Day 1 - Day 6: Bleeding/menstruation Period

🪷 Day 14: Ovulation

▨ Not recommended for M.U.M.™

▨ **Best Time to perform M.U.M™.** On Ovulation day, it is ideal to perform (self) M.U.M.™ 30-60 minutes before sexual intercourse.

**Important Note:** Do not perform the Massage AFTER insemination or intercourse

▨ Fertile Period

▨ M.U.M.™ is permissible only when confirmed not pregnant.

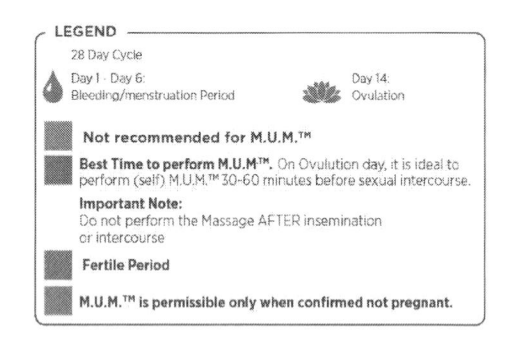

**Table 2**: 28 Days Menstrual Cycle Sample based on the Four Seasons of the Menstrual Cycle

Both Professional M.U.M™ Fertility Massage or Self M.U.M.™ Fertility Massage need to be done in a calm and relaxed environment. You may have them done in the morning immediately after you wake up, or in the evening after a warm bath. The latter is recommended. You should avoid having the massage performed between activities or during work, especially if you are rushed for time. Having said that, it is at least better to perform the massage then not at all. As recommended in Table 1, M.U.M.™ can be done at all times, except for when you are having your menses or if you are pregnant.

As with any massage therapy, you need to satisfy the recommended number of treatments hours in order to see positive results. As with M.U.M.™, regardless if you are trying to get pregnant naturally or with assistance, we recommend that you incorporate M.U.M.™ as part of your daily health regime. We recommend our clients to perform at least 20 hour of massage[40] on their abdomen with a combination of Professional M.U.M™ Fertility Massage and Self M.U.M.™ Fertility Massage, in order to yield positive results.

Self M.U.M.™ Fertility Massage should only be

---

[40] Wurn et al., *Treating female infertility and improving IVF pregnancy rates with a manual physical therapy technique.*

done after a tutorial session with a trained M.U.M.™ instructor. Through reading this book or the Part II: Self M.U.M.™ Fertility Massage, Step by Step Techniques with Illustration, although you may understand the concept of how to perform the massage, you may not be able to evaluate or execute, the proper techniques of the massage, considering a practical learning is required for techniques like applying the right pressure, proper hand positioning or properly identifying the landmarks on your body.

## Contraindications to Performing Malay Uterus Massage™ by Salwa Salim

In all cases, it is always best to get your doctor's approval before proceeding with any treatments outside your doctor's medical care. Below are the contraindications when it is not recommended to perform M.U.M.™:

- Immediately after meals
- During menses
- Suffering from pain or cramps
- During your ovulation period
- With a full bladder
- After sexual intercourse (insemination of sperm into the uterus)

## Fertility Massage for Women

- Suspected pregnancy
- Pregnant
- Immediately after normal delivery or after C-section
- Any health issues or medical conditions
- After any assisted conception procedure (IVF/IUI) — discontinue after implantation of embryo
- IUD implant
- Fever, sore throat or any form of infection
- Active infection in the abdomen or pelvis
- Pelvic Inflammatory Disease (P.I.D)
- After any surgery or medical procedures

Salwa Salim

## Locating Reproductive Organs Based on Body Landmarks

Below are the three major landmarks that you need to know. Your M.U.M.™ instructor will guide you on how to physically locate these landmarks.

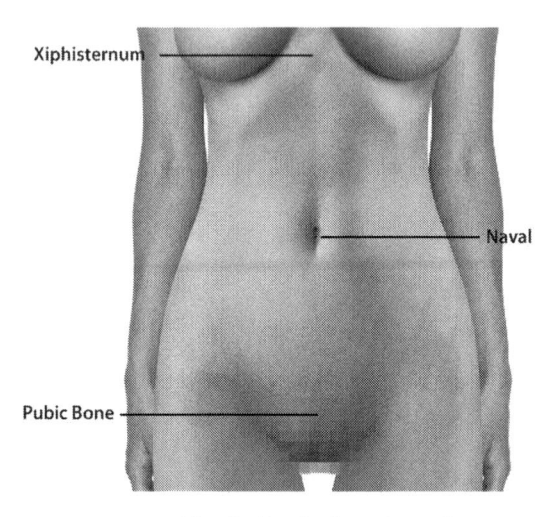

**Fig 8: Body Landmarks**

Fertility Massage for Women

## Locating the Pubic Bone

The pubic bone is an important landmark to identify, as it is used as an indicator to locate where other organs are. By looking at your navel, draw a straight line downwards, and as soon as you touch the hard bony parts, right above the pubic hairline, that is your pubic bone. The other way to locate it is by placing your palm flat on your tummy, placing both thumbs on your navel and letting your index fingers meet symmetrically down, creating a triangle. You will be able to feel the start of the pubic bone.

## Locating the Uterus

The uterus starts right above the pubic bone and extends above up to 7.5 centimeters in length. The average size, weight, shape and location of the uterus may vary; however, the starting point is typically at the pubic bone. In order to perform (Self) M.U.M.™, it is not important for you to know the position or angle of your uterus (anteverted, retroverted, axial, etc.). All you need to know is the approximate location of where the uterus lies. For thinner bodies, if your uterus is in the right position, when you press the tips of your finger inwards right above the pubic bone with an empty bladder, you may feel the base of the uterus as strong fibrous tissues, with a little bounce. In some cases, you may not feel it due to the muscles or layer of fat that may be in the way.

## Locating the Ovaries

The two ovaries are located on either side of the uterus and can be determined by drawing a straight line 10 centimeters down from the navel, and then approximately 7 centimeters distally/outwardly (right and left).

The other way is similar to finding your pubic bone by forming a triangle with your thumb and fingers with your hands flat on your tummy where the tip of your last fingers lie; the pinkies are where your ovaries lie.

# PART IV

## BENEFITS OF M.U.M.™ FERTILITY MASSAGE

# CHAPTER 4.1

## General Benefits

This chapter highlights the benefits of M.U.M.™ Fertility Massage as a whole, focusing on the conditions that may lead to infertility. M.U.M.™ does not only improve the overall health of the uterus, it also addresses specific issues or conditions that are related to female reproductive organs. The attention of this chapter is on the benefits of M.U.M.™ to overcome specific conditions stated below. As a caution, M.U.M.™ is not meant to diagnose or treat any of these conditions, nor is this meant to replace the advice of your medical practitioner.

### Improvement of Blood Circulation and Lymphatic Drainage

A "cold" uterus or cervix describes one that does not receive good blood circulation. When there is not

## Fertility Massage for Women

enough blood circulation in the lower abdomen, it results in a poor supply of fresh oxygenated blood to the reproductive organs and build-up of toxic waste, which may be one of the causes infertility. M.U.M.™ Fertility Massage improves circulation in many ways, as described in the following paragraphs.

Firstly, massage over the abdominal areas helps overall blood circulation. The increased supply of oxygenated and well-nourished blood not only helps with the building of healthy blood vessels of the endometrium layer, but also for all other organs. This includes the ovaries for more quality eggs, strengthening of the ligaments supporting the reproductive organs, and also non-reproductive organs, such as the large and small intestines, stomach and liver. This in turn promotes the removal of old stagnant cells, and blood and tissues that are still lingering in the uterus at a more efficient rate so it does not cause much damage to the organs.

As M.U.M.™ improves blood circulation to the pelvic areas, it inadvertently stimulates the lymphatic drainage. The stimulation of lymphatic drainage helps to speed up the removal of all toxic waste material that may cause lymphatic congestion. This results in reduced acidity in the tissue by helping drain waste material. This will further cause a positive chain reaction in educed inflammation and optimized nerve sensitivity to the pelvic area. This is particularly beneficial for women who lead sedentary lifestyles, where they sit for more than six hours a day. Our body was not designed for such a lifestyle. Sitting for long periods of time causes the bent area, like a kink in a straw, incidentally at the reproductive organs juncture of the pelvic area where reduction of blood flow forms in that particular position.

## Regulating Hormones

The communication of hormones in the body between the different organs, including pituitary, hypothalamus, ovaries and uterus is called the feedback loop. M.U.M.™ Fertility Massage helps with controlling the levels of hormones produced when being stimulated; thus, helps in the healthy and clear communication resulting in a healthier hormonal balance.

Since hormones are transported through the bloodstream, having a healthy blood circulation results in having more balanced hormones, as it regulates the menstrual cycle that is vital for fertility. The uterus requires a clear and direct line of communication with the brain so that the uterus is able to access the right amount of progesterone and estrogen. This creates an optimum, healthy environment for a healthy egg to ripen, ovulate, transit and be implanted.

## Breaking Down Scar Tissue/Adhesion

Adhesion is a natural process of the building of fibrous bands internally or externally between any structures of tissues and organs as part of the recovery period from surgeries, inflammation or trauma. Adhesion, also called scar tissues, naturally makes these connections between surfaces that, under normal circumstances, are not connected. Adhesion can also be caused by toxin buildup or high blood sugar levels; therefore, uterus massage is the only non-invasive method to date that can either prevent these adhesions from building up, which may cause blockages or, help break down these adhesions that have already been formed internally in the reproductive organs or surrounding structures. The physical manipulation in breaking the links formed from these adhesions will not only help to get rid of these unwanted waste products, but will not create tightness and tension between any surfaces.

One of the more common conditions that M.U.M.™ helps treat is blocked fallopian tubes. A clear fallopian tube is crucial for the passage of the sperm to meet the egg. So having a blocked fallopian tube is a major malfunction that stops the sperm from reaching the egg and is the cause of many cases of infertility. If these blockages are caused by adhesions, the only non-invasive way to deal with this issue is through massage. Studies have shown the effectiveness of these types of massage over the fallopian tube to help with the condition. M.U.M.™ is very effective in using physical manipulation to loosen and break down these fibrous adhesions. Once these adhesions are broken down, they are easily eliminated. Regular massages ensure that you are not allowing the buildup to recur.

Salwa Salim

## Cleansing and Detoxifying

Cleansing is an extension of circulation. Improved circulation promotes the removal of toxic waste accumulated in the uterus and which was not gotten rid of during menstruation. A healthy menstrual discharge should comprise of bright red and un-clotted blood. This demonstrates a healthy womb where blood is immediately discharged out of the body the moment it disintegrates itself from the endometrium. Dark reddish to brown blood, especially having a foul smell, indicates that it remained stagnant and was retained in the body before it was discharged. M.U.M.™ will help to remove any of this "old" blood, dead endometrium cells, or tissues that are stagnant and may still be stuck to the uterine walls.

In cases where the woman had previous pregnancies, regardless if she had a live birth, a miscarriage, abortion or even a stillborn baby, the uterus may have remnants of pregnancy tissues and blood present, months after the procedure. M.U.M.™ usually accompanied with heat therapy, is effective in helping rid all of the old blood, dead cells and necrotic pregnancy tissue that may still be present after the procedures. M.U.M.™ will promote the expulsion of any unwanted stale materials out of the body for a healthy reproductive system for a regular menstrual cycle.

# CHAPTER 4.2

## Uterus

## Reinstating Misaligned, Tilted or Prolapsed Uterus

As shown in Chapter 1.4, there are four ligaments that hold the uterus in place, including the round ligaments on either lateral side (front and back ligaments). The uterus is said to be suspended freely in the pelvic bowl and capable of moving freely forwards or backwards. If the rectum and bladder were empty, in most normal cases, these ligaments would hold up the uterus to form a right angle with the vagina, forming an anteverted position in the pelvic bowl. About 20% of women have naturally different variations where the most occurring position is the retroverted[41]. Although

---

[41] Theron, J.P. (1963). The retroverted uterus, an evaluation of the

there is no clear evidence linking the variation of the positions of the uterus to the causes of infertility, these uncommon positions may be the cause of menstrual issues or painful intercourse.

Regardless of the natural position of the uterus, there are many reasons why and how the uterus can be misaligned, tilted, prolapsed, or simply displaced from its original position. Hippocrates famous for his teachings in medicine who lived in the 2nd Century, described the uterus as the wondering womb. He wrote a description of the ability of the womb to be out of place from a fixed position in the body. There are many possible causes for the uterus to be displaced, considering the uterus is suspended freely in the pelvic bowl, being held together by many different ligaments with many adjacent organs directly impacting it.

## Possible Causes of Misaligned, Tilted or Displaced Uterus:

- Repeated pregnancy

---

Moschowitz Operation, South African Journal of Obstetrics and Gynecology, 68, 68-74.

## Fertility Massage for Women

- Poor care during pregnancy, delivery and postnatal period
- Weak core pelvic muscles, or poor strengthening and conditioning of lower back muscles
- Overweight
- Vigorous exercise
- Compression by fecal impacted intestines
- Lack of circulation or scar tissues
- Past pelvic surgeries
- Carrying heavy burdens immediately pre or during menstruation, or too soon after childbirth
- Injury to sacrum
- Chronic constipation
- Poor alignment of pelvis
- Carrying young children on the hip for a long time
- Emotional armoring
- Straining during bowel movement
- Prolonged and improper use of tight corsets
- Standing or sitting for very long hours
- Sudden loss of massive weight, especially pelvic fats, which help hold up the uterus

## **Possible Signs & Symptoms of a Misaligned, Tilted or Displaced Uterus:**

- Dark brownish or dark red menstrual blood
- Painful periods and/or during ovulation
- Irregular menstrual cycles and ovulation
- Miscarriages and difficult pregnancies
- Endometriosis /endometritis
- During menopause period and menopausal symptoms
- Infertility issues
- PMS depression with menstruation
- Ovarian cysts
- Uterine fibroids or polyps
- Abnormal uterine bleeding
- Bladder yeast infection
- Displaced or prolapsed uterus or bladder
- Leaking or frequent urination (incontinence)
- Bladder infection
- Sexual concerns, like loosened vagina, or discomfort with a feeling of a small mass falling out of your vagina
- Hemorrhoids

- Varicose veins
- Tired, weak legs
- Numb legs and feet

The ideal uterus position for a childbearing woman is anterverted, where in its natural state, it is able to move around quite freely with no restrictions. It is far more common than many women realize, at one point of time in their life, to have their uterus displaced out of its original position. Some cases can be very severe, where the misalignments or displacement may cause conditions such as a prolapsed uterus, which needs medical intervention i.e. major surgery. M.U.M.™ is a non-invasive technique that does not require surgery to reinstate the uterus if it is misaligned, displaced or presented with a mild prolapse. Through M.U.M.™, it helps to loosen ligaments and the surrounding organs and break down any adhesions or scar tissues within the ligaments that is causing the unnatural tightness to one side of the ligaments, and hence gently pushes up the uterus with repeated, slow and gentle physical manipulation.

There have been many incidences where M.U.M.™ clients reported feeling mobile and lighter immediately after just one session. The correct positioning of the uterus can give a sense of balance, where the center of the lower abdomen is strengthened, allowing for more flexibility and a more active lifestyle.

## Endometriosis

Endometriosis is a medical condition where the uterus lining is found growing abnormally outside of the uterus. Endometrial cells may travels outside of the uterine cavities and attach themselves to other parts of the reproductive organs such as the ovaries, pelvic ligaments, fallopian tubes, bladder, bowels, etc. All endometrial tissues then build up and bleed during menses. However since these happens outside of the uterus, the blood is unable to escape therefore the surrounding tissues and organs may sticks together. This can cause scarring, tubal blockages, ovulation problems, pelvic pain and abnormal menstrual cycles.

Some of the more common symptoms for women having endometriosis is painful menstrual period before and during menses, pain during and/or after sexual intercourse, lower back pain during menses, diarrhea during menses, pain while urinating and defecating during menses.

M.U.M.™ helps with pain management normally associated with endometriosis. Massage will help with breaking down of the adhesions and scarring present within the abdomen, and removal of these dead cells and toxic buildups to improve circulation in the abdomen areas. The physical manipulation of massage can help to disintegrate the abnormal links and scarring created between structures, and also clear the passages in the fallopian tubes, or break. This also helps with estrogen clearance, where it increases the circulation into the uterus

## Fibroids

Uterine fibroids are non-cancerous, benign tumors or growths, having different pathology functions, sizes and forms. It may occur anywhere in any layer of the uterus, or even on the linings of the uterus, which may or may not cause pain or heavy, painful periods. They are easily detected by an ultrasound and if they are large, they may exert pressure on the bladder and bowels, and even distend the abdomen.

Fibroids may even have their own blood supply, so one of the greatest benefits of massage is the ability to break down adhesions surrounding and supporting the fibroids, bringing circulation back to the pelvic area, since the uterus already gets as little as only 5% of blood supply[42]. Especially with large uterine fibroids where it may be located in an area causing compression on the blood supply that may result in compromising circulation to the reproductive organs and the surrounding organs.

---

[42] Lefkowitz M.R & Fant M.B. (2005). *Women's Life In Greece And Rome*, London, JHU Press, 248.

# CHAPTER 4.3

## Ovaries

### Polycystic Ovarian Syndrome (PCOS)

This is one of the more common reasons for infertility affecting up to 5-10% of childbearing women[43]. PCOS is caused by a hormonal imbalance that disrupts the ovulation, where it occurs less frequent than normal, affecting fertility. Women usually suffer from irregular cycles, weight gain, acne and excessive hair growth, as a result of this syndrome.

Scar tissue and congestion caused by numerous undeveloped cysts are broken down and eliminated

---

[43] Trivax, B. & R Azziz. (2007). Diagnosis Of Polycystic Ovary Syndrome. *Clinical Obstetrics And Gynecology*, no. 50: 168-177.

through the lymphatic system and an increase in blood circulation. M.U.M.™ is effective for common ovarian issues, such as ovarian cysts and polycystic ovarian syndrome. By increasing the circulation through massage, it brings fresh oxygenated blood to the ovaries, delivering nutrients and hormones to the developing follicles. This process also speeds up the negative feedback loop between the ovaries and pituitary gland to maintain the hormonal balance and better ovarian function.

PCOS is one of the more common cases in our program, and is hard to isolate the reasons for the success of our clients' pregnancies. Some underwent M.U.M.™ in conjunction with other treatments, and some independently. The first common feedback we get is that their menstrual cycle starts to get more and more regular and predictable. Following the massage, there are clients reporting the increase in the number and size of healthy eggs to be extracted for their IVF procedures. Others had successfully gotten pregnant within just a month of starting our program.

## Premature Ovarian Failure (POF)

POF is a condition of premature menopause, where women's periods may either stop completely or became very irregular. The ovaries stop producing estrogen and eggs, making natural conception unlikely.

As mentioned previously, the control of hormonal balance may be strengthened by uterus massage. With a good hormonal feedback loop system, an increase in circulation with fresh oxygenated and nutrient rich blood supply, sped up elimination of toxins, helping in the overall health of the eggs. The effectiveness in clearing congestions, reducing of inflammation, promoting hormonal balance, and increasing circulation; thus, nutrition to your eggs may encourage a normal function of ovarian systems preventing abnormal, premature eggs of the ovaries.

# CHAPTER 4.4

# Fallopian Tube

## Fallopian Tube Occlusion

The fallopian tube may be occluded due to many reasons. One of the more common reasons is where the occlusion are reversible is when the fallopian tubes are twisted or blocked by adhesion, scar tissues, or dead cells. This creates a blockage and prevents the natural route of the egg to meet the sperm for fertilization, and reaching the uterus. To date, uterus massage is the only available, non-invasive technique that can help clear any blocked fallopian tubes. The massage techniques help to reduce inflammation and break down adhesions, clearing the tubes for the egg to travel to the uterus. Many women come to us with this issue of having one or both fallopian tubes blocked and are eager to perform M.U.M.™, considering the positive results from research that proves how massage can be an effective method for clearing fallopian tube occlusion[44].

---

[44] Wurn et al., *Treating Fallopian Tube Occlusion with A Manual Pelvic Physical Therapy.*

# CHAPTER 4.5

## Surrounding Organs

The other organs that will be involved in M.U.M.™ Fertility Massage are the stomach, liver and intestines, which are adjacent to the reproductive system. Massaging the liver is beneficial in removing toxins and hormones out of the body, whereas massaging the stomach and intestines helps in digestion, as it moves the feces that may be stuck or impacted.

While massage increases circulation to the digestive system, it also boosts immunity. Eighty percent of our immune system is activated by the digestive system. Immunity, digestion, and fertility are all interrelated. There are some views linking an imbalanced immune system to unexplained infertility, as well as the 80% of unexplained miscarriages[45]. Indirectly, a bad digestive system leads to a digestive disorder, leading to poor absorption of nutrients.

Considering that the uterus rests at right angles on top of the bladder, incontinence is a very common issue amongst women who had given birth or had undergone a miscarriage/abortion. M.U.M.™ is mostly known for repositioning the uterus in the original position, and one of the most prevalent symptoms M.U.M.™ has relieved is incontinence. M.U.M.™ is a popular treatment for postnatal women, for this reason.

## Constipation & Irritable Bowel Syndrome

These are the two most common digestive problems that may directly or indirectly be the cause of, or affecting the neighboring organs adjacent to it i.e. the reproductive systems. Part of the M.U.M.™ Fertility Massage involves massaging the upper and lower abdominal area to encourage the movement of waste and fecal matter along the digestive tract. Massage helps to manually push the waste and fecal matter out of the

---

[45] Beer A. E, Kantecki J. & Jane Reed. 2006. *Is Your Body Baby-Friendly?*. Houston, TX: AJR Pub.

body, relieving constipation by promoting bowel movements. Especially if fecal matter that is stuck in a particular crease in the large intestines for a longer period of time, turning it unnaturally hard, massage can help to dislodge it and move it along. This helps with the overall strengthening of the intestines to greatly relieve constipation, release wind or bloating, and also promotes the proper function of the bowel movement which affects the normal functions of the adjacent reproductive system.

# CHAPTER 4.6

## Emotional Release

Ever wondered where terms such as "butterflies in my stomach" or "feel sick in my stomach" or "gut wrenching" came about? Our body holds onto our negative emotions, especially stress, worries, and fears in the abdominal areas. Storing negative feelings in our body triggers negative hormonal responses, which may be detrimental to the body, especially during the fertile period. Emotional healing is necessary in order to release pent-up emotions that may be stored in the body, creating a block. This inhibitor is a direct link on how our emotions can affect our fertility, especially in the cases of unexplained infertility.

M.U.M.™ Fertility Massage helps to release these stored negative emotions that may cause the blockage and disintegrate the bad emotions that may have been the cause of an otherwise healthy and functioning reproductive system. Fertility massage gently eases the tension in the body. Combined with guided meditations or visualizations, women can center themselves and feel a connection with their uterus and visualize themselves seeing a baby bump. I have personally experienced women in the midst of a soothing massage, bursting into tears and emotions while performing the massage.

# PART V ANNEX

RESEARCH STUDIES ON MASSAGE, REPRODUCTIVE HEALTH & INFERTILITY IN WOMEN

# Massage Improves Pregnancy Rates and Improves Successful IVF

## Research Title: Treating female infertility and improving IVF pregnancy rates with a manual physical therapy technique

Wurn, B., Wurn, L., Roscow, A., King, R., Heuer, M., & et al. (2004). Treating female infertility and improving IVF pregnancy rates with a manual physical therapy technique, *MedGenMed*, *6*(2), 51.

Mechanical adhesions are among the most established causes of female infertility. These adhesions are described as connective tissue deposits that form in response to surgical or inflammatory insults. These fibrous tissues often adhere to certain structures, e.g., pelvic organs, muscles, etc., and hence, the name "adhesions". They have also been implicated as a concurrent problem among women diagnosed with pelvic inflammatory disease, endometriosis polyps, and pelvic spams.

The results of recent studies on the benefits of manual pelvic therapy in the management of infertility, due to pelvic adhesion, have been promising. Pelvic massage was shown to cause micro-failures in intra-abdominopelvic adhesions and effectively break them apart. As such, subsequent studies among women diagnosed with infertility and who underwent manual physical therapy show that their conception rates increased, reaching as much as 46%.

Guided by these trends, two studies were conducted between 1998 and 2002 to further evaluate the benefits of manual pelvic therapy in treating female infertility caused by tubal occlusion.

## Study I: To determine the benefits of manual physical manipulation on women with adhesions-related infertility

Fourteen women, who were diagnosed with infertility caused by confirmed or suspected pelvic adhesions, were recruited. Among these women, 92% had either an infectious or inflammatory disease, while others had abdominopelvic trauma or abdominopelvic surgeries.

The subjects of the study were later monitored and allowed to complete at least 20 hours of manual pelvic manipulation. They received no other treatment for infertility. Outcomes for this study were measured through successful natural intrauterine pregnancy rates.

Fertility Massage for Women

Data obtained from the study showed that about 10 or 71% of all 14 women had successfully and naturally conceived after the treatment. The study ultimately showed that strategic manual pelvic therapy could serve as a useful adjunctive therapy for the treatment of adhesion-related infertility among women.

## Study II: To determine the benefits of manual physical therapy on women who attempted to conceive after IVF

This time, for the second stage of the aforementioned study, a total of 25 women were recruited. The primary consideration for inclusion was the women's inability to conceive after 12 months of unprotected sexual intercourse. Additional inclusion criteria included the women's intent to have IVF in the next 15 months, using their own embryos and progressing embryo transfer into the ART process.

After the selection process, the women underwent manual pelvic therapy and completed at least 10 hours of therapy. This time, rather than evaluating the natural intrauterine pregnancy rates, outcomes for study II were measured using in-vitro fertilization (IVF) pregnancy rates.

Using the expected odds ratio, it was found that 47.7% of those who opt to transfer from natural to IVF pregnancy finally bear children within 15 months after the treatment. Both studies intensify the evidence base, supporting the benefits of manual pelvic therapy in treating female infertility, secondary to tubal occlusion.

Indeed, manual pelvic therapy can improve treatment outcomes for women who wish to bear children naturally or otherwise.

# Massage Improves Women's Reproductive Health

## Research Title: Treating fallopian tube occlusion with a manual pelvic physical therapy

Wurn, B., Wurn, L., Roscow, A., King, R., Heuer, M., & et al. (2008). Treating fallopian tube occlusion with a manual pelvic physical therapy, *Alternative Therapies, 14*(1), 18-23.

Pelvic adhesions have been shown to impair female fertility and reduce success rates for IVF. These adhesions are caused either by previous abdominal surgeries, endometriosis, previous infection, or ectopic pregnancy. Following the surgical or inflammatory insult, the body forms micro-adhesions, which later turn into adhesions and ultimately into scars.

More recent studies have shown, however, that manual therapy, or more specifically, sustained pelvic physical therapy, creates structural changes in pelvic adhesions, altering connective tissue mobility and length. It was further theorized that mobilization of these soft tissues disrupts collagenous cross-links, which are the primary culprits for female reproductive dysfunction.

In this study, a retrospective analysis was done in examining the ability of pelvic physical therapy in re-opening fallopian tubes, which have been completely occluded by adhesions. The study was done with a sample of 28 women diagnosed with infertility, secondary to complete occlusion of the fallopian tubes. These women were also treated for concurrent abdominopelvic dysfunctions, e.g., dyspareunia, dysmenorrhea, pelvic pain, etc.

These women were exposed to a total of 20-hour sessions of manual physical therapy intended to improve connective tissue mobility and address pain caused by pelvic adhesions. Included in this therapy was the direct manipulation of deep pelvic structures, including the fallopian tubes and even the uterine ovarian ligaments, the peritoneum, and other areas in surrounding organs. Efficacy was objectively determined by two outcome measures: 1) reopening of one or both fallopian tubes, as confirmed by imaging tests; and, 2) non-artificial intrauterine pregnancy rates occurring in the next two years from the start of the manual pelvic therapy.

Approximately 61% of patients were diagnostically found to have improved fallopian tube latency within just a month after undergoing therapy, and among these women, 9 or 53% had successful non-artificial pregnancy. Hence, although spontaneous reopening of truly occluded fallopian tubes has not been established, this study substantiates the value of using manual pelvic therapy as an adjunct to the current gynecologic management through surgery for tubal occlusion.

Salwa Salim

# Research Title: Decreasing dyspareunia and dysmenorrhea in women with endometriosis via a manual physical therapy: Results from two independent studies

Wurn, B., Wurn, L., Patterson, K., King, R., & Scharf, E.S. (2011). Decreasing dyspareunia and dysmenorrhea in women with endometriosis via a manual physical therapy: Results from two independent studies. *Journal of Endometriosis*, *3*(4), 188 – 196.

Retrograde menstruation, or the reflux of the endometrial products of menstruation, which subsequently implant on structures other than the uterus, e.g., the fallopian tube, ovaries, peritoneal structures, etc., is considered as the most plausible etiology of endometriosis. Implantation of the endometrium to structures outside the uterus leads to a number of painful and disturbing disease conditions, such as dyspareunia, dysmenorrhea and pelvic adhesions.

Fortunately, after a series of animal-based experiments, manual pelvic therapy was found to reduce abdominopelvic adhesions related to endometriosis. In fact, in another study, a non-invasive and site-specific therapy known as the "Wurn Technique" was also found to improve natural intrauterine pregnancy rates, enhance IVF pregnancy, and relieve dyspareunia among women diagnosed with infertility. It was further found that sustained mechanical manipulation of adhesions disrupt connective tissue bonds and subsequently, alter adhesion, mobility and strength.

With this, two independent studies were conducted to assess the benefits of the Wurn Technique to relieve pain during intercourse and dysmenorrhea among women diagnosed with endometriosis through a retrospective and a prospective study, respectively. To this end, a sample of women surgically diagnosed with endometriosis, were evaluated following a total of 20-hour long therapy sessions using the Wurn technique. This technique is a site-specific and non-invasive manual physical therapy strategically designed to disrupt adhesions and relieve restrictions caused by connective tissues in both the abdomen and pelvic floor. To evaluate the Wurn Technique's effectiveness, the Female Sexual Function Index and the Mankoski Pain Scale were used six weeks after therapy. The index and scale were used to evaluate the benefits of the Wurn Technique on dysmenorrhea and pain during sexual intercourse, respectively.

Indeed, this study further intensifies the value of a non-invasive and site-specific manual physical therapy as an adjunctive treatment for women with dysmenorrhea and dyspareunia. Moreover, these positive outcomes warrant further investigation in order to further substantiate the efficiency of this non-invasive and, hence, more convenient treatment modality for dyspareunia and dysmenorrhea.

# Relationship Between Stress and Infertility

## Research Title: Preconception stress increases the risk of infertility: Results from a couple-based prospective cohort study—the LIFE study

Lynch, C. D., R. Sundaram, J. M., Maisog, Sweeney, A.M., & Louis, G. (2014). Preconception stress increases the risk of infertility: Results from a couple-based prospective cohort study-The LIFE study. *Human Reproduction 29* (5), 1067-1075.

The relationship between stress and reproduction has been quite controversial; however, since its conception, no study has ever successfully linked stress to fertility. This study represents the first study to ever demonstrate a significant relationship between stress and reproduction in the United States. As its primary objective, the study aimed to collect tangible evidence to elucidate the relationship between stress and fertility.

A total of 501 couples were recruited in this prospective cohort study. The levels of cortisol and alpha-amylase in the saliva were measured, and the two were used as biomarkers for stress in the study. Both biomarkers were measured twice, once in the morning after enrollment as baseline values, and another the morning after the women's first menstrual period during the study hoping to measure the women's stress levels after realizing that they failed to get pregnant. Moreover, as a measure of fertility, the time-to-pregnancy (TTP) was measured in cycles. Couples were followed-up within a 12-month period.

Among the 501 couples recruited for the study, 100 dropped out, leaving only 401, or 80% of the couples to complete the study protocol. Within the follow-up period, a large number, or exactly 347 (87%) of the women, became pregnant, while only 54 (13%) failed to get pregnant. Based on the levels of alpha-amylase in the saliva, it was found that women who had the highest salivary alpha-amylase level had a significant (29%) reduction in fecundity, i.e., longer TTP, as compared with women with low salivary alpha-amylase levels. Further statistical analysis also showed that such decreases in fecundity could be translated to as much as a two-fold risk for infertility. Cortisol levels, however, were found to be unrelated to the risk for infertility. Results of the study imply that stress-reduction could prove to be highly beneficial to women who wish to bear children.

Being the first study to successfully demonstrate a tangible association between stress and fertility in the U.S., the study proves to be highly beneficial in the current efforts of treating infertility. Indeed, the study has its limitations, i.e., collection of samples of saliva were only done twice, high dropout rate, and it was unable to collect repeated data for the perceived stress questionnaire; however, it is undeniable that the study was able to pave the way for further research studies. All in the hopes of explaining and accurately describing how stress affects women's ability to conceive and bear children. This is critical, especially in the backdrop of increasing incidence of infertility across the United States and in many other countries.

# Research Title: Stressful life events are associated with a poor in-vitro fertilization (IVF) outcome: a prospective study

Ebbesen, S.M.S., Zachariae, R., Mehlsen, M.Y., Thomsen, D., Hojgaard, A., Ottosen, L., Petersen, T., & H.J. Ingerslev. (2009). Stressful life events are associated with a poor in-vitro fertilization (IVF) outcome: A prospective study. *Human Reproduction 24*(9), 2173-2182.

Recent studies have slowly uncovered the relationship between stress and fertility; however, this study conducted back in 2009 attempted to establish the impact of stress on the success rates of in-vitro fertilization (IVF). IVF has fairly recently gained much interest among couples that wish to conceive. Indeed, this study proved to be a very interesting one as it was the first to touch on the concept of improving IVF conception outcomes. The primary objective of the study was to describe the relationship between negative life events, i.e. stressful events occurring 12 months prior to the procedure and IVF success rates.

The study recruited a total of 837 women with a mean age of 31.2 years. At the outset, the subjects were tasked to complete a List of Related Events (LRE). They answered questionnaires that determined the subjects' perceived stress levels and identified depressive symptoms. Another parameter measured in the study was pregnancy, which was defined through a pregnancy test. Pregnancy tests were considered positive when the serum Beta hCG levels were more than 20 IU, two weeks after the transfer of the embryo. Furthermore, clinical pregnancy was also detected by identifying a live intrauterine pregnancy via transabdominal or transvaginal ultrasound.

A total of 18 cases had missing data and were excluded from the data analysis. Overall, 819 cases were included in the data analysis. Multiple regression analysis was done to test the results, and it was found that women who failed in IVF reported more negative life events as compared to those who had fewer negative life events. Hence, like other studies conducted to correlate stress and fertility, stress is also associated with negative IVF outcomes. In terms of depressive symptoms, total number of life events on LRE and perceived level of stress however, independent sample T-test has shown no significant difference between successful and unsuccessful IVF patients.

Taking the study further, the researchers went on to correlate the number of oocytes harvested during oocyte retrieval with stress, and found the same correlation. Also, specific life events were identified to be highly correlated with IVF success. Among those identified are experience of violence and illness in the family or of the patient.

IVF is now becoming a highly accepted and extremely hopeful treatment for couples wishing to get pregnant. Indeed, this study has been vastly innovative as it provides relevant information on how to improve IVF success rates. The study has clearly shown how high levels of stress prevent women from successfully conceiving following IVF. Hence, stress-reduction techniques are implicated as beneficial treatment modalities prior to commencing with IVF.

# Relationship Between Relaxation and Improved Fertility

## Research Title: The effect of relaxation techniques to ease the stress in infertile women

Valiani M. et al. (2005). The Effect of Relaxation Techniques to Ease The Stress In Infertile Women, *Iranian Journal of Nursing and Midwifery Research*, 15 no. 4: 259.

As a valuable addition to modern fertility research, this study explored the benefits of relaxation techniques in reducing stress and subsequently improving women's chances of conceiving. Study after study has shown how high levels of stress is verifiably linked with the inability to conceive.

The association between stress and infertility is thought to be caused by the psychological effects of the couples' failure to conceive. Such may lead to increased tension between couples and subsequently further increase stress as they deal with sadness, despair, frustration, anger and distress. In fact, other women have reported that infertility is the most stressful event that they have experienced in their entire existence. It is for these reasons that stress-reduction techniques are highly acknowledged in infertility treatment.

The researchers conducted a semi-experimental and a clinical trial study to explore the benefits of relaxation techniques in reducing stress levels among infertile women. To this end, a total of 76 reproductive-age women diagnosed with primary infertility and who were under assisted reproductive techniques (ART), either in vitro fertilization (IVF) or intra-cytoplasmic sperm injection (ICSI), were recruited for the study. Women who fit the inclusion and exclusion criteria were randomly placed under two groups, i.e., intervention and control groups. At the outset, the participants' levels of stress were obtained through Newton's infertility stress questionnaire. After which, participants under the intervention group received relaxation techniques for a total of 12 sessions. Stress questionnaires were subsequently distributed after embryo transfer and after two weeks, before conducting a pregnancy test.

Results of the study were analyzed using independent samples T-test. Baseline stress scores were found to be similar between the two groups, showing no significant difference between the stress scores of the intervention and control groups at the beginning of the study. However, stress scores were found to be significantly different after the implementation of relaxation techniques, wherein those who did not receive any treatment reported higher stress scores as compared to the intervention group.

The study was able to successfully validate the benefits of relaxation techniques in reducing stress scores of women diagnosed with infertility. Indeed, these relaxation techniques can be used as an adjunct to ARTs to further improve conception outcomes. Then again, it would have been to everyone's advantage if the researchers took the study further by comparing the pregnancy outcomes of those who received relaxation techniques to those who did not. Still, the results of the study are considered no less favorable in improving current efforts of treating infertility.

Salwa Salim

# Research Title: Stress reduces conception probabilities across the fertile window: evidence in support of relaxation

Louis, G. M., Lum, K., Sundaram, R., Chen, Z., Kim, S., Lynch, C., Schisterman, E., & Pyper, C.(2011). Stress reduces conception probabilities across the fertile window: Evidence in support of relaxation. *Fertility And Sterility 95* (7), 2184-2189.

The high prevalence of infertility in the today's society has ignited recent advances in infertility research. A number of modern lifestyle factors have been identified to increase the risk for infertility, including cigarette smoking, obesity, drinking alcoholic beverages, among others. Further, perceived psychological stress has also been implicated as an important factor in successfully conceiving. This is evidenced by studies that show infertile women finally bearing children after child adoption or after receiving stress-reduction therapies.

It is the objective of this study to explore the relationship between stress levels, quantified through two biomarkers, salivary alpha-amylase and cortisol levels, and human fecundity, described as time-to-pregnancy. This was done using a prospective cohort study conducted in the United Kingdom.

## Fertility Massage for Women

The study comprised 374 reproductive age women with regular menstrual cycles and who were attempting to bear children for less than three months. To improve the researchers understanding of their experiences, the participants were asked to complete a diary to note their menstrual cycles, sexual intercourse and document lifestyle behaviors such as smoking, drinking, etc. Moreover, to monitor reproductive hormones (i.e. estrogen and LH), the respondents were also asked to test their urine with a fertility monitor beginning day 6 until day 20 of their menses. Further, salivary alpha-amylase and cortisol levels were measured on day 6 of their menses, as well.

After careful statistical analysis, data showed that increased salivary alpha-amylase and not cortisol levels were associated with negative fecundity outcomes. It is estimated that the odds of failing in the respondents' attempts to conceive is 85%, if elevated alpha-amylase levels are detected in the saliva. A significant decline in the probability of conceiving was observed among women who had salivary alpha-amylase levels found in the upper quartiles, as compared with women with salivary alpha-amylase levels in the lower quartiles.

The study has successfully revealed objective information on the relationship between stress and fertility. While the study was unable to specifically identify the exact salivary alpha-amylase levels to be at-risk for decreased fecundity, the study was certainly able to highlight the role of salivary alpha-amylase levels as a potentially vital biomarker for predicting success in infertility treatment. Moreover, among the strengths of this study was the detailed description of the various methods and statistical tools used for the objectives of this study. The researchers have gone through great lengths to extract related information regarding stress and infertility. Indeed, stress-reduction techniques can prove to be strongly advantageous for women who want to conceive.

# Reducing Stress Through Massage

## Research Title: Cortisol decreases and serotonin and dopamine increase following massage therapy

Field T. et al. (2005) Cortisol decreases and serotonin and dopamine increase following massage therapy. *Int J Neurosci* 115, no. 10 (2005): 1397-1413.

The study explored the biochemical effects of massage therapy in a population of individuals suffering from depression, pain syndromes, autoimmune-related diseases, as well as pregnancy, and age and job-related stress. Biochemical markers reviewed in the studies include cortisol, serotonin and dopamine.

Cortisol is known as the "Stress Hormone," as it is found to increase during stressful conditions, and such ultimately negatively affects the body's immune defenses. As such, this hormone has been used as a biomarker for stress and is often measured before and after massage therapy sessions. Another biochemical marker used is serotonin. It is a CNS-activating neurotransmitter measured in urine samples.

Serotonin is the primary hormone controlled in various depressive states. Dopamine has similar CNS activating effects as serotonin, and regulating these two (serotonin and dopamine) may be beneficial in improving depressed states and the associated stressful outcomes.

Studies that measured cortisol after administering massage therapy sessions showed significant decreases in both urine and salivary cortisol, ranging from 19% to 45% in urine samples and between 10% and 37% in salivary samples. Moreover, the levels of serotonin and dopamine were assayed in the urine. In several studies, an average increase of 31% was reported for dopamine and while an average increase of 28% was noted for serotonin following massage therapy. Further, among women with eating disorders, there was a noted increase in dopamine levels up to as much as 42% after undergoing massage therapy sessions. Other studies have also confirmed the positive effects of massage therapy for those with pain syndromes. Studies have shown that massage therapy effectively reduces perceived pain levels as a result of reduced pain, depression and anger. These studies provide valuable evidence on the benefits of massage therapy for relieving stress and other conditions that lead to stress.

The studies have effectively shown how stress induces various biochemical changes in the body, and how massage therapy effects relief at a biochemical level. Unfortunately, the study's primary drawback was the lack of any detailed description of the methods used in the review of related literature. Nonetheless, it was able to bring to light, important and perhaps even groundbreaking research studies on the benefits of massage therapy in reducing stress.

Salwa Salim

# Research Title: Physiological adjustments to stress measures following massage therapy

Oraska, A., Pollini, R., Boulanger, K., Brooks, M., & Teitlebaum. L. (2010). Physiological adjustments to stress measures following massage therapy: A review of the literature. *Evidence-Based Complementary And Alternative Medicine, 7* (4), 409-418.

The study reviews recently conducted studies that focused on stress and massage therapy. Stress was described as the disruption in the body's physiologic equilibrium as a result of psychological, emotional, or physical distress. Massage therapy, on the other hand, was defined as the act of manipulating soft tissues to produce physiologic effects to the body. This study attempts to synthesize the large and vastly variable studies conducted that attempts to ascertain the impact of massage therapy on various physiologic measures of stress.

The study searched peer-reviewed journals published in four online databases namely: MEDLINE, CINAHL, Psych INFO and Massage Therapy Foundation. This was done using the keyword "stress," combined with the following terms: "massage," "physiotherapy," "bodywork," and "manual therapy". These search terms initially generated a total of 1032 related articles, which were subsequently reviewed for relatedness to the topic. Ultimately, after screening the articles for relevance and quality, only 25 articles were found to have complied with all the inclusion criteria set in the study. Among these studies, physiologic parameters, such as hormones, catecholamines, blood pressure and heart rate were used to measure the impact of massage therapy were evaluated.

Among the 25 studies, massage therapy was administered in a period of about 20 to 30 minutes, two times a week, in a period of five weeks. Moreover, measurement of physiologic parameters was done prior to the first session and after one or over a series of massage therapy sessions.

From 25 related articles, 89% of the studies showed that salivary cortisol has a significant relationship to stress; however, one study failed to establish such a relationship. Urinary cortisol, on the other hand, was used to measure the effects of massage therapy after multiple treatments. Three of the nine related studies were able to show a significant correlation, and one study found that three massage therapy sessions are unable to produce significant outcomes. Studies that used plasma cortisol, on the other hand, were not comprehensive enough to be included in the literature review. Apart from cortisol, catecholamines were also used as a physiologic parameter. Review of such studies shows no change in serum and urine epinephrine and norepinephrine levels.

Also, in determining levels of stress, blood pressure, and heart rate were also used. Eight studies were found to correlate the effects of stress on blood pressure. Among the eight identified studies, three reported significant findings. Among these studies, the noted change in blood pressure was minimal, ranging between 2 to 12mmHg. Finally, heart rate was evaluated as a physiologic parameter of stress in 11 studies. Like blood pressure, there are few studies that report significant change, and those who reported significant changes; the changes were also minimal, about 3 to 6 beats per minute right after a single massage therapy session.

After thorough review of the vast literature on the topic of massage therapy and stress, there still is no consensus on the benefits of massage therapy on different stress-related physiologic parameters. Nonetheless, the benefits of massage therapy to reducing stress levels prove to be a very fertile ground for future research.

# GLOSSARY

| Foreign Word | Translation |
| --- | --- |
| *Bidan/ Bidan Kampung / Mak Bidan* | Midwife/Village Midwife |
| *Chi Nei Tsang* | A treatment modality of healing touch originating from Taoist Chinese |
| *Ganggang* | Vaginal steam therapy for women |
| *Jamu* | Herbal medicine |
| *Jiwa, Raga, Sukma* | Mind, body, soul |
| *Kampung* | Village |
| *Mandian* | Herbal Bath |
| *Pijat* | Massage |

| | |
|---|---|
| *Qi/Ki* | A concept of life force, natural energy or energy flow |
| *Qi Gong* | Practice of aligning breath with body and mind for health, meditation and marital arts training |
| *Ratus (See Ganggang)* | Vaginal steam therapy for women |
| *Reiki* | A treatment where there is transference of Ki through palm healing or hands on healing touch |
| *Tai Qi* | Chinese martial arts practiced for defense and health benefits |
| *Tui Na* | Hands on body treatment where *tui* means push and *na* means lift/squeeze |
| *Tukang Urut/Tabib Urut* | Massage therapist, masseur, masseuse |

## Fertility Massage for Women

| | |
|---|---|
| *Tungku/Tuam* | A form of treatment using a heated stone/metal/steel applied on the body |
| *Kong Fu* | A form of Chinese marital arts |
| *Sengkak* | A specialized abdominal massage technique for women to help with reproductive health |
| *Urut* | Massage |
| *Urut Batin* | Manhood Massage |
| *Merian, Penyawa, Peranak, Peranakan, Rahim,* | Uterus/womb |

# BIBLIOGRAPHY

Aflakseir, A., & Zarei, M. (2013). Association between coping strategies and infertility stress among a group of women with fertility problems in Shiraz, Iran. *Journal Of Reproduction And Infertility, 14 (4)*, 202-206.

American Society for Reproductive Medicine. (2012). Medication for inducing ovulation, Patient Information Series, *American Society for Reproductive Medicine*. Retrieved from: http://www.asrm.org/uploadedFiles/ASRM_Content/Resources/Patient_Resources/Fact_Sheets_and_Info_Booklets/ovulation_drugs.pdf, 8-9

Barakbah, A. (2007), Ensiklopedia Perbidanan Melayu. Cheras, Kuala Lumpur: Utusan Publication & Distributor.

Beck, M. (2010). *Theory & practice of therapeutic massage* (5th ed.). Clifton Park: Delmar Cengage Learning.

Braun, M., & Simonson, S. (2005). *Introduction to massage therapy*. Philadelphia: Lippincott Williams & Wilkins.

Louis, G. M., Lum, K., Sundaram, R., Chen, Z., Kim, S., Lynch, C., Schisterman, E., & Pyper, C.(2011). Stress reduces conception probabilities across the fertile window: Evidence in support of relaxation. *Fertility And Sterility 95* (7), 2184-2189.

Calver, R. (2002). The history of massage: An illustrated survey from around the world. Vermont: Healings Arts Press.

Center for Human Reproduction, (2015), Unexplained Infertility, *Centre for Human Reproduction*. Retrieved from: www.centerforhumanreprod.com/infertilityedu/causes/unexplained/

Chuthaputti A, & Boonterm, B. (2010). *Traditional medicine in ASEAN*. Bangkok: Bangkok Medical Publisher.

Clare, B. (2015). *Fertility massage therapy (*1st ed.). Mayfair, London: Fertility Massage Therapy & Training.

Clay, R. (2006). Does stress hinder conception? The relationship between mental state and fertility is a complex one. *American Psychological Association,37 (8)*. Retrieved from: http://www.apa.org/monitor/sep06/stress.aspx

Coleman, J., & Nonacs, R. (2015). Infertility, assisted reproduction and mental health, MGH Center for Women's Mental Health, *Massachusetts General Hospital*. Retrieved from:

http://womensmentalhealth.org/resource/patient-support-services/infertility-assisted-reproduction-and-mental-health/

Deka, P. K. (2010). Psychological aspects of infertility. *British Journal of Medical Practitioners, 3* (3), a336.

Domar, A. D. (2007). Coping with the Stress of Infertility, Fact Sheet Series, Fact Sheet 15, Infertility & Stress. *RESOLVE: The National Infertility Association*, Retrieve from: http://familybuilding.resolve.org/site/DocServer/15_Coping_with_the_Stress_of_Infertility.pdf?docID=5705

Domar, A. D. (2014). Depression and infertility: treatment considerations, Managing Infertility Stress, *RESOLVE: The National Infertility Association*. http://www.resolve.org/support/Managing-Infertility-Stress/depression-and-infertility-treatment-considerations.html

Domar, A. D. (2015). Will massage help me get pregnant?, *Baby Centre*. http://www.babycenter.com/404_will-massage-help-me- get-pregnant_1411676.bc

Domar, A. D. (2015c). What truly is the relationship between stress and IVF outcome?, *The Domar Center for Mind & Body Health*. Retrieve from: www.domarcenter.com/blog/2011/03/what-truly-is-the-relationship-between-stress-and-ivf-outcome-2/

Ebbesen, S.M.S., Zachariae, R., Mehlsen, M.Y., Thomsen, D., Hojgaard, A., Ottosen, L., Petersen, T., & H.J. Ingerslev. (2009). Stressful life events are associated with a poor in-vitro fertilization (IVF) outcome: A prospective study. *Human Reproduction 24*(9), 2173-2182.

European Society for Human Reproduction and Embryology, (2006), Behavioural therapy can restore ovulation in infertile women. *European Society for Human Reproduction and Embryology*. Retrieve from: http://www.sciencedaily.com/releases/2006/06/060621084306.html

Field, T., Hernandez-Reif, M., M.D. Diego, S. Schanberg, & C. Kuhn. (2005). Cortisol decreases and serotonin and dopamine increase following massage therapy. Int J Neurosci, 115(10), 1397-1413.

Gerber, R., & M. Williams (2002). *Geography, culture, and education*. Dordrecht: Kluwer Academic Publishers.

Gilman, S.L. (1993). *Hysteria beyond freud*. Berkeley: University of California Press.

Gupta, S., Ghulmiyyah, J., Sharma, R., Halabi, J., & Agarwal, A. (2014). Power of proteomics in linking oxidative stress and female infertility. *Biomed Research International*, 1-26.

Hou, W., Pai-Tsung, C., Tun-Yen, H., Su-Ying, C., & Yen, C. (2010). Treatment effects of massage therapy in depressed people. *The Journal of Clinical Psychiatry, 71*(7), 894-901.

Human Fertilisation & Embryology Authority. (2014). What is intrauterine insemination (IUI) and how does it work?, *Human Fertilisation & Embryology Authority*. Retrieve from: http://www.hfea.gov.uk/IUI.html

Jensen, J.T., & Mishell, D. (2012). Family planning: Contraception, sterilization, and pregnancy termination. *Comprehensive Gynecology, 215*.

Keng, S. (2005). Malaysian midwives' views on postnatal depression. *British Journal of Midwifery, 13*(2), 78-86.

Kit, L., Kick, G., & Ravindran, J. (1997). Incidence of postnatal depression in Malaysian women. *Journal of Obstetrics and Gynaecology Research, 23*(1), 85-89.

Larsen, U. (2005). Research on infertility: Which definition should we use? *Fertility and Sterility, 83*(5), 846-852.

Lee, J. & Hopkins, V. (2015). Infertility: Getting pregnant and staying pregnant. *Virginia Hopkins Test Kit. Retrieve from:* http://www.virginiahopkinstestkits.com/infertility.html

Lefkowitz, M. & Fant, M. (2005). *Women's life in Greece and Rome*. London: JHU Press.

Lentz G. M.(2012) Primary and secondary dysmenorrhea, premenstrual syndrome, and premenstrual dysphoric disorder: etiology, diagnosis, management. In: Lentz G.M., Lobo R.A., Gershenson D.M., Katz V.L., eds. *Comprehensive Gynecology*. 6th ed. Philadelphia, PA: Elsevier Mosby: chap. 36.

Lewis, H., & Lewis, M. (1972). *Psychosomatics: How your emotions can damage your health*. New York: Viking Press.

Lobo, R. (2012). Infertility: etiology, diagnostic evaluation, management, prognosis. In: Lentz G.M., Lobo R.A., Gershenson D.M., Katz V.L., eds. *Comprehensive Gynecology*. 6th ed. Philadelphia, PA: Elsevier Mosby: chap. 41.

Lynch, C. D., R. Sundaram, J. M., Maisog, Sweeney, A.M., & Louis, G. (2014). Preconception stress increases the risk of infertility: Results from a couple-based prospective cohort study-The LIFE study. *Human Reproduction 29* (5), 1067-1075.

Mascarenhas, M. N., Flaxman, S.R., Boerma, T., Vanderpoel, S., & and Stevens, G. (2012). National, regional, and global trends in infertility prevalence since 1990: A systematic analysis of 277 health surveys', *Plos Med, 9* (12).

Mayor, C. A., Rounds, J., & Hannum, J. (2005). A meta-analysis of massage therapy research. *Psychological Bulletin, 130*(1), 3-18.

Mercier, J., & , and Miller, K. (2013). Mercier therapy helps infertile women achieve pregnancy. *Midwifery Today With International Midwife,* 105, 40, 68.

Ministry of health of republic of Indonesia. (2007). *National policy on traditional medicines.* Jakarta: Ministry of Health R.I..

Moraska, A., Pollini, R., Boulanger, K., Brooks, M., & Teitlebaum. L. (2010). Physiological adjustments to stress measures following massage therapy: A review of the literature. *Evidence-Based Complementary And Alternative Medicine , 7* (4), 409-418.

Moyer, C. (2008). Research section editorial: Affective massage therapy. *International Journal Of Therapeutic Massage And Body Work, 1*(2), 3-5.

Mumford, K. (2004). The stress response, psychoeducational interventions and assisted reproduction technology treatment outcomes: A meta-analytic review. (Graduate Theses and Dissertation, University of South Florida, Scholar Commons, 2004), 32 – 27.

National Center for Complementary and Alternative Medicine. (2008) Complementary, alternative, or integrative health: What's in a name?. *National Center for Complementary and Integrative Health,* Publication

D347. Retrieve from: https://nccih.nih.gov/sites/nccam.nih.gov/files/CAM_Basics_What_Are_CAIHA_07-15-2014.2.pdf

Nelson, A. & Gellar, P. (2012). Coping with fertility treatment: Infertility-related stress and social support among women receiving in-vitro fertilization. *Gender Medicine, 9*(1).

Oates, M., Cox, J., Neema, S., Asten, P., Glangeaud-Freudenthal, N., Figueiredo, B., & Gorman, L. et al. (2004). Postnatal depression across countries and cultures: A qualitative study. *The British Journal of Psychiatry, 184*(46), s10-s16.

Pettman, E. (2007). A history of manipulative therapy. *Journal of Manual & Manipulative Therapy, 15*(3), 165-174.

Rapaport, M., Schettler, P., & Bresee, C. (2012). A preliminary study of the effects of repeated massage on hypothalamic–pituitary– adrenal and immune function in healthy individuals: A study of mechanisms of action and dosage. *The Journal Of Alternative And Complementary Medicine,,18*(8), 789-797.

Reich, W. (1972). *Character Analysis*. New York: Farrar, Straus and Giroux.

Resolve.org, (2015), What Are My Chances of Success With IVF, RESLOVE: *The National Infertility Association*, Retrieve from: http://www.resolve.org/family-building-options/ivf-art/what-are-my-chances-of-success-with-ivf.htm

Rice, A. D. (2013). Manual physical therapy for non-surgical treatment of adhesion-related small bowel obstructions: Two case reports., *J. Clin. Med, 2*(1), 1-12.

Rutstein, S. and Shah, I. (2004). DHS Comparitive Reports No 9. Infecundity, Infertility and Childlessness in Developing Countries. ORC Marco, World Health Organisation. Retrieve from: http://www.who.int/reproductivehealth/topics/infertility/DHS-CR9.pdf

Sarrel, P., & DeCherney, A. (1985). Psychotherapeutic intervention for treatment of couples with secondary infertility, *Fertility and Sterility, 43*(6), 897-900.

Shapiro, C. (2010). New research on stress and infertility. *Psychology Today*, Retrieve from: https://www.psychologytoday.com/blog/when-youre-not- â€¨expecting/201008/new-research-stress-and-infertility

Stephanie, (2013). The retroverted and retroflexed uterus: From front to back (Well, mostly, back). [Web Log Post]. Feminist Midwife. Retrieve from: http://www.feministmidwife.com/2013/12/04/the-retroverted-and-retroflexed-uterus-from-front-to-back-well-mostly-back/#ixzz35ABkh3kP

Theron, J.P. (1963). The retroverted uterus, an evaluation of the Moschowitz Operation, *South African Journal of Obstetrics and Gynecology, 68*, 68-74.

Thiering, P., Beaurepaire, J., Langeluddecke, P., Kellow, J., & Tennant, C. (1993). Mood state as a predictor of treatment outcome after in- vitro fertilization/embryo transfer technology (IVF/ET), *Journal of Psychosomatic Research, 37*(5), 481-491.

Uba, L. (1992). Cultural barriers to health care for Southeast Asian refugees, *Public Health Rep, 107*(5), 544–548.

Valiani, M., Abediyan, S., Ahmadi, S., Pahlavanzadeh, S., & and Hassanzadeh, A. (2005). The effect of relaxation techniques to ease the stress in infertile women, *Iranian Journal of Nursing and Midwifery Research, 15*(4), 259.

Van Der Giessen, M. (1990). Psyche and soma, *Massage Therapy Journal, 29*(30), 66-82.

Vickers, A. & Zollman, C. (2001). Massage therapies, *Western Journal of Medicine, 175*(3), 202-204.

Wasser, S., Sewall,G., & Soules, M. (1993). Psychosocial stress as a cause of infertility, *Fertility and Sterility, 59*(3), 685- 689.

Wheldon, J. (2015). Stress may be causing infertility in women, *Mail Online*. Retrieve from:

http://www.dailymail.co.uk/health/article-391616/Stress-causing-infertility-women.html

World Health Organisation (WHO). (2015). Infertility definitions and terminology, Sexual and reproductive health, *World Health Organization*. Retrieve from: http://www.who.int/reproductivehealth/topics/infertility/definitions/en/

World Health Organisation (WHO). (2013).WHO Traditional Medicine Strategy, 2014-2023. *Hong Kong, China: World Health Organization*, Retrieve from: http://apps.who.int/iris/bitstream/10665/92455/1/9789241506090_eng.pdf

Wurn, B., Wurn, L., Roscow, A., King, R., Heuer, M., & et al. (2004). Treating female infertility and improving IVF pregnancy rates with a manual physical therapy technique, *MedGenMed*, *6*(2), 51.

Wurn, B., Wurn, L., Roscow, A., King, R., Heuer, M., & et al. (2008). Treating fallopian tube occlusion with a manual pelvic physical therapy, *Alternative Therapies*, *14*(1), 18-23.

Wurn, B., Wurn, L., Patterson, K., King, R., & Scharf, E.S. (2011). Decreasing dyspareunia and dysmenorrhea in women with endometriosis via a manual physical therapy: Results from two independent studies. *Journal of Endometriosis*, *3*(4), 188 – 196.

Zegers-Hochschild, F. (2006). The ICMART glossary on ART terminology, *Human Reproduction, 21*(8).

Zegers-Hochschild, F., Adamson, G., de Mouzon, J., & et al. (2009). International committee for monitoring assisted reproductive technology (ICMART) and the World Health Organization (WHO) Revised glossary of ART terminology, *Fertility And Sterility, 92*(5), 1520-1524, 1522.

# INDEX

abdominal sacral technique 68

abortion 78, 104, 118

adhesion 8, 10, 26, 55, 66-68 ,77, 80, 102, 103, 109-110, 111, 115, 123-125, 127, 128, 130, 131

Arvigo Technique Mayan Abdominal Therapy (ATMAT) 60

assisted reproductive technology (ART) 6

bladder 20, 22, 25, 59, 65, 94, 97, 105, 108, 110, 111, 118

body basal temperature xv, 84-85

cervical 5, 66

cervical mucus xv, 38, 85

cervix 6, 20, 22, 24-26, 29, 36, 100

*Chi Nei Tsang* 51-52

circulation 10, 52, 60, 79, 100-102,104, 107,110-111,113-114,117

complementary and alternative medicine (CAM) 46, 148

constipation 22, 52, 107, 118, 119

cramp 52, 54, 60, 94

diarrhea 52, 110

depression 10, 17, 51-52, 56, 73, 108, 145-146

egg 3, 6, 16, 20, 24-25, 31, 35-37, 39, 83-85, 88-90, 101-103, 113-115

emotion 13-15, 51-52, 120-121

emotional 4, 13-17, 41-42, 44, 52, 61, 65, 68, 107, 120, 148

endometrial 36, 38-39, 90, 110, 130

endometriosis 5, 26, 65, 80, 108, 110, 123, 127, 130-131

endometrium 5, 36-39, 79, 87-88, 90, 101, 104, 130

estrogen 20, 31, 35-38, 102, 111, 113, 143

fallopian tube 16, 24-25, 28, 36-37, 65, 67, 80, 89, 103, 110, 115-116, 127-128, 130

- blocked fallopian tube 8, 67, 80, 103, 115

- fallopian tube occlusion 115-116, 127

fertile body xiv, 3, 15

fertile body model xiv, xviii, 85

fertilization 6, 17, 25, 31, 33, 36-37, 39, 85, 90, 115, 125, 136, 140

fibroids 5, 60, 108, 111

follicle 31, 35-36, 113

follicle stimulating hormones (FSH) 31

follicular 31, 35, 83

*ganggang* 54-55, 58, 79

heat compression 55, 78

heat therapy 70, 74, 78, 104

herbal ball 78

herbal bath 58

hormonal xv, 5-6, 10, 57, 102, 112-114, 120

hormones vii, 4, 10, 20, 24, 31, 35-80, 102, 113, 117, 143, 149

in vitro fertilisation (IVF) 6-8, 17, 67, 81, 89, 95, 113, 123, 125, 131, 136-138, 140

infection 95, 108, 127

infertility x, xi, xiv, xvi, 2-9,12-18, 25-26, 43-44, 47-49, 53-54, 56-58, 66-67, 71, 75, 80, 82, 93, 100-101, 103, 106, 108, 112, 117, 120, 122-125, 128, 131, 133-135, 139-142, 144

- unexplained infertility 5, 6, 12-13, 17, 117, 120, 168, 65, 101, 103, 114-115

inflammation 26, 65, 101, 103, 114-115

intestines 19-20, 22, 101, 107, 117, 119

intra uterine insemination (IUI) 7, 67, 81, 89, 95

irritable bowel 54, 74, 118

*jamu* 57-58

ligaments 10, 25, 28, 30, 33, 49, 76-78, 101, 105-106, 109-110, 128

liver 20, 52, 101, 117

luteal 37, 83

luteinizing hormones (LH) 31, 35-36, 143

lymph 60, 69, 78

lymph nodes 60, 78

lymphatic 10, 28, 49, 52, 100-101, 113

Malay xi, xii, xiii, xvii, xix, 53-58, 70-72, 74-75, 77, 79, 81, 94

- Malay archipelago xiii, 53
- Malay culture 53, 58
- Malay language xiii, 53, 72
- Malay midwifery 71
- Malay traditional medicine xii, 55-56, 71
- Malay traditional postnatal care 56, 73
- Malay traditional practice 75, 79

mental 4, 13, 15, 17, 41, 42, 44, 61

midwife/midwives xi, 72-73

midwifery 53, 72-73, 139

mind and body xv, 12-13, 17, 62

mind-body 7, 13, 15

miscarriage 55, 71, 78, 104, 108, 118

menopausal xvi, 74, 80, 108

menopause 108, 113

menses 26, 87, 88, 90, 93-94, 110, 143

menstrual xvi, 25, 31-33, 36-39, 52, 57, 74, 78, 80, 82-92, 102, 104, 106, 108, 110, 113, 134, 143

muscles 3, 9-10, 16, 25, 49, 61, 68, 76-78, 97, 107, 123

ovarian 28, 33, 35, 83, 108, 112-114, 128

ovaries 10, 24-25, 28, 31-32, 35, 65, 77, 83, 88, 98, 101-102, 110, 112-114, 130

ovulate 5, 31, 102

ovulation 31, 33, 36-37, 39, 80, 83,-85, 89, 94, 108, 110, 112

ovulatory 5, 36

pain 7, 26, 28, 43, 59, 63, 65-67, 69, 94, 110-111, 128, 131, 145-146

pelvic inflammatory diseases (PID) 26, 65, 95, 123

pelvis10, 25, 65-66, 78, 81, 95, 107

physical therapy 63-64, 66, 123-125, 127, 128, 130-131

physiotherapy 26, 63, 148

polycystic ovary syndrome (PCOS) 112

polyp 60, 123

postnatal xvi, 53-56, 71, 74, 80, 107, 118

postnatal care 53, 56, 71-73, 80

postnatal depression 56, 73

postnatal massage 54

postnatal period 107

premature ovarian failure (POF) 113

premenstrual syndrome 52, 159

progesterone 32, 37-38, 88, 102

proliferative 38, 83

*qi* 48-49, 51-52

reproductive x, xiii, xvi, 2, 4, 6, 9-10, 15, 19-20, 23-24, 27, 30, 33, 50, 52, 65, 68-69, 71, 74-76, 78, 80, 82-83, 96, 100-104, 110-111, 117-119, 121, 127, 140, 143

- reproductive health x, xiii, 71, 74, 80, 127

- reproductive organ 4, 10, 15, 20, 24, 52, 76, 80, 96, 100-103, 110-111

- reproductive system xiii, 2, 9-10, 19, 23-24, 27, 30, 33, 50, 69, 71, 78, 80, 82-83, 104, 117-119, 121

relaxation 9, 15, 17-18, 43, 139-142

*ratus* 58, 152

*reiki* 61-62

sacrum 10, 29, 76, 78, 107

scar 66, 77, 102-103, 107, 109, 112, 115, 127

scar tissues 77, 103, 107, 109, 115

scarring 8, 55,110

secretary 38

*sengkak* 54, 57, 74-77, 153

spiritual 15, 42, 44, 51, 58-59, 65

stillborn 104

stomach 20, 52, 102, 117, 120

stress xv, xx, 5, 8,-10, 13, 16-17, 44, 52, 69, 80, 120, 130, 133-150

tension 10, 13-14, 52, 68-69, 76, 103-104, 121, 139

traditional medicine xii, 41-42, 44-45, 48, 54-56, 59, 71-72

traditional, complimentary & alternative medicine (TCAM) x, xii, 45-47, 52

traditional Chinese medicine (TCM) 48, 50-52

*tuam* 54-55, 78

*tungku* 54-55, 78

uterine 5, 25, 28-29, 33, 38, 60, 83, 89, 104, 108, 110, 111, 128 uterus xii, xiii, xiv, 6, 10, 20, 22, 24-26, 28-29, 31-32, 37-39, 48, 54-55, 57, 59-60, 65, 70, 72, 74-77, 81, 83, 87-88, 90, 94, 97-98, 100-111, 114-115, 118, 121, 130

- misaligned, tilted, displaced uterus 77, 105-106, 108-109

- prolapsed uterus 74, 77, 105-106, 108-109

uterus lining 37, 110

uterus heat therapy 70, 74, 78

*urut* xiii, xix, 53-54, 57, 73

*urut batin* 54

vagina 22, 24, 26, 28, 55, 79, 105, 108

vaginal 54-55, 58, 70, 74, 79, 80

vaginal steam therapy 70, 74, 79-80

womb xiii, xiv, 104, 106

World Health Organization (WHO) xii, 44, 53, 72

# ABOUT AUTHOR

Salwa Salim is a women's natural reproductive health expert. Her previous experiences as a healthcare professional, working with Singapore's leading hospitals and clinics, has equipped her with vast knowledge and understanding of the reproductive functions and diseases of women. As the founder of Mummy's Group, her companies provide pregnancy, postpartum and fertility services. In addition, through the Mummy's Education & Outreach Program, Salwa is active in the community locally and internationally providing training and lectures.

Fertility Massage for Women:

Introducing Malay Uterus Massage (M.U.M.) ™ by Salwa Salim

PART II: Self M.U.M.™ Fertility Massage — Step by Step Technique with Illustration

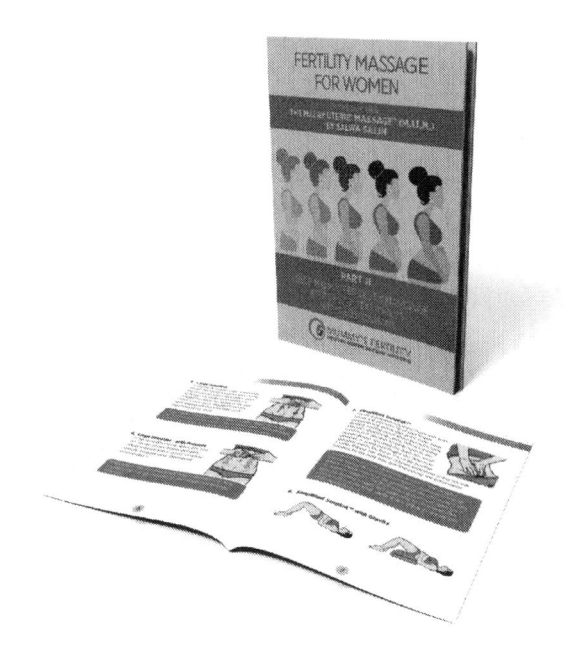

For more information, visit www.MummysFertility.com

Printed in Poland
by Amazon Fulfillment
Poland Sp. z o.o., Wrocław